T0200005

Standardized Evaluation in Clinical Practice

Review of Psychiatry Series
John M. Oldham, M.D., M.S.
Michelle B. Riba, M.D., M.S.
Series Editors

Standardized Evaluation in Clinical Practice

EDITED BY

Michael B. First, M.D.

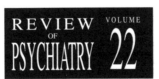

No. 2

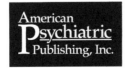

Washington, DC
London, England

Note: The authors have worked to ensure that all information in this book is accurate at the time of publication and consistent with general psychiatric and medical standards, and that information concerning drug dosages, schedules, and routes of administration is accurate at the time of publication and consistent with standards set by the U. S. Food and Drug Administration and the general medical community. As medical research and practice continue to advance, however, therapeutic standards may change. Moreover, specific situations may require a specific therapeutic response not included in this book. For these reasons and because human and mechanical errors sometimes occur, we recommend that readers follow the advice of physicians directly involved in their care or the care of a member of their family.

Books published by American Psychiatric Publishing, Inc., represent the views and opinions of the individual authors and do not necessarily represent the policies and opinions of APPI or the American Psychiatric Association.

Copyright © 2003 American Psychiatric Publishing, Inc.
07   06   05   04   03   5   4   3   2   1

ALL RIGHTS RESERVED
Manufactured in the United States of America on acid-free paper
First Edition

Typeset in Adobe's Palatino

American Psychiatric Publishing, Inc.
1000 Wilson Boulevard
Arlington, VA 22209-3901
www.appi.org

The correct citation for this book is

First MB (editor): *Standardized Evaluation in Clinical Practice* (Review of Psychiatry Series, Volume 22, Number 2; Oldham JM and Riba MB, series editors). Washington, DC, American Psychiatric Publishing, 2003

Library of Congress Cataloging-in-Publication Data
Standardized evaluation in clinical practice / edited by Michael B. First.
      p. ; cm. — (Review of psychiatry ; v. 22)
   Includes bibliographical references and index.
   ISBN 1-58562-114-5 (alk. paper)
    1. Psychological tests. 2. Behavioral assessment. 3. Psychodiagnostics. I. First,
      Michael B., 1956– II. Review of psychiatry series ; 22, 2.
   [DNLM: 1. Mental Disorders—diagnosis. 2. Diagnosis, Differential. 3. Process
   Assessment (Health Care). 4. Risk Factors. 5. Severity of Illness Index. 6. Suicide,
   Attempted—psychology. WM 141 S785 2003]
   RC469.S68 2003
   616.89′075—dc21

                                                                    2002043868

British Library Cataloguing in Publication Data
A CIP record is available from the British Library.

Contents

Contributors

Monica Ramirez Basco, Ph.D.
Associate Professor, Department of Psychiatry and Division of Psychology, University of Texas Southwestern Medical Center at Dallas, Dallas, Texas

Michael B. First, M.D.
Associate Professor of Clinical Psychiatry, Columbia University; Research Psychiatrist, New York State Psychiatric Institute, New York, New York

Batsheva Halberstam, B.A.
Research Worker, Department of Neuroscience, New York State Psychiatric Institute and Columbia University, New York, New York

Kathy L. Henderson, M.D.
Manager, South Central VA Health Care Network Mental Health Product Line, Little Rock, Arkansas

Christopher P. Lucas, M.D., M.P.H.
Assistant Professor of Clinical Psychiatry, Columbia University and New York State Psychiatric Institute, New York, New York

J. John Mann, M.D.
Professor of Psychiatry and Radiology, Columbia University; Chief, Department of Neuroscience, New York State Psychiatric Institute, New York, New York

Rudolf H. Moos, Ph.D.
Senior Research Career Scientist and Professor, Center for Health Care Evaluation, Veterans Affairs Health Care System and Stanford University, Palo Alto, California

John M. Oldham, M.D., M.S.
Professor and Chair, Department of Psychiatry and Behavioral Sciences, Medical University of South Carolina, Charleston, South Carolina

Maria A. Oquendo, M.D.
Associate Clinical Professor of Psychiatry, Columbia University; Director of Clinical Studies, Department of Neuroscience, New York State Psychiatric Institute, New York, New York

Michelle B. Riba, M.D., M.S.
Clinical Professor and Associate Chair for Education and Academic Affairs, Department of Psychiatry, University of Michigan Medical School, Ann Arbor, Michigan

Robert Rosenheck, M.D.
Director, Northeast Program Evaluation Center, VA Connecticut Healthcare System, West Haven, Connecticut; Professor of Psychiatry and Public Health, Yale Medical School, New Haven, Connecticut

Mary Schohn, Ph.D.
Chief, Clinical Office of Behavioral Health, VISN 2, Buffalo, New York

William W. Van Stone, M.D.
Associate Chief for Psychiatry, Veterans Affairs Central Office, Washington, D.C.

Mark Zimmerman, M.D.
Associate Professor, Department of Psychiatry and Human Behavior, Brown University School of Medicine, Rhode Island Hospital, Providence, Rhode Island

Introduction to the Review of Psychiatry Series

John M. Oldham, M.D., M.S.
Michelle B. Riba, M.D., M.S., Series Editors

2003 REVIEW OF PSYCHIATRY SERIES TITLES

- *Molecular Neurobiology for the Clinician*
  EDITED BY DENNIS S. CHARNEY, M.D.
- *Standardized Evaluation in Clinical Practice*
  EDITED BY MICHAEL B. FIRST, M.D.
- *Trauma and Disaster Responses and Management*
  EDITED BY ROBERT J. URSANO, M.D., AND
  ANN E. NORWOOD, M.D.
- *Geriatric Psychiatry*
  EDITED BY ALAN M. MELLOW, M.D., PH.D.

As our world becomes increasingly complex, we are learning more and living longer, yet we are presented with ever more complicated biological and psychosocial challenges. Packing into our heads all of the new things to know is a daunting task indeed. Keeping up with our children, all of whom learn to use computers and how to surf the Internet almost before they learn English, is even more challenging, but there is an excitement that accompanies these new languages that is sometimes almost breathtaking.

The explosion of knowledge in the field of molecular neurobiology charges ahead at breakneck speed, so that we have truly arrived at the technological doorway that is beginning to reveal the basic molecular and genetic fault lines of complex psychiatric diseases. In *Molecular Neurobiology for the Clinician,* edited by Dr. Charney, Dr. McMahon (Chapter 2) outlines a number of genetic discoveries that have the potential to affect our clinical practice in important ways, such as validating diagnostic systems and

---

disease entities, improving treatment planning, and developing novel therapies and preventive interventions. Examples of these principles are illustrated in this book as they apply to addictive disorders (Chapter 4, by Dr. Nestler), schizophrenia (Chapter 3, by Dr. Gilbert and colleagues), psychiatric disorders of childhood and adolescence (Chapter 1, by Drs. Veenstra-VanderWeele and Cook), and mood and anxiety disorders (Chapter 5, by Dr. Gould and colleagues).

Increased precision and standardization characterizes not only the microworld of research but also the macroworld of clinical practice. Current recommendations regarding standardized assessment in clinical practice are reviewed in *Standardized Evaluation in Clinical Practice,* edited by Dr. First, recognizing that we must be prepared to reshape our diagnostic ideas based on new evidence from molecular genetics and neurobiology, as well as from the findings of clinical research itself. In Chapter 1, Dr. Basco outlines a number of problems inherent in routine clinical diagnostic practice, including inaccurate or incomplete diagnoses, omission of comorbidities, and various sources of bias, and an argument is made to train clinicians in the use of a standardized diagnostic method, such as the *Structured Clinical Interview for DSM* (SCID). Similar problems are reviewed by Dr. Lucas (Chapter 3) in work with child and adolescent patients, and a self-report diagnostic assessment technique, the Computerized Diagnostic Interview Schedule for Children (C-DISC), is described. The C-DISC is reported to have the advantages of enhancing patients' abilities to discuss their concerns and enhanced caretaker satisfaction with the intake interview.

Similarly, Dr. Zimmerman (Chapter 2) underscores the importance of developing a standardized clinical measure with good psychometric properties that could be incorporated into routine clinical practice, presenting data suggesting the value of one such system, the Rhode Island Methods to Improve Diagnostic Assessment and Services (MIDAS) project. Dr. Oquendo and colleagues (Chapter 4), in turn, review the critical issue of the use of standardized scales to enhance detection of suicidal behavior and risk of suicide in individual patients. The challenge to establish the cost-effectiveness of standardized assessment methodology in clinical practice is illustrated by the efforts in the U.S. Department of Veterans Affairs system, described by Dr. Van Stone and colleagues (Chapter 5), to train clinicians in the use of the Global Assessment of Functioning (GAF) scale, and to incorporate it into the electronic medical record.

In *Trauma and Disaster Responses and Management,* edited by Drs. Ursano and Norwood, a compelling case is made by Dr. Bonne and colleagues (Chapter 1) of the fundamental interconnectedness between lifelong biological processes in humans and animals, and the environment. The relevance of studies using animal models to our understanding of posttraumatic stress disorder and other stress syndromes has become increasingly important, elucidating the functional neuroanatomy and neuroendocrinology of stress responses. This growing research database proves compelling when contemplating the human impact of major disasters such as the Oklahoma City bombing, described by Dr. North (Chapter 2), the effect of the World Trade Center tragedy and other disasters on developing children, described by Drs. Lubit and Eth (Chapter 3), and the potential and actual impact of bioterrorism on individuals and large populations, reviewed by Dr. Ursano and colleagues (Chapter 5). The need for early intervention, articulated by Dr. Watson and colleagues (Chapter 4), becomes increasingly clear as we learn more, which we must, about trauma and its effects.

As we learn more about many things, we make progress, but always with a cost. We are getting better at fighting illness and preserving health, hence we live longer. With longer life, however, comes new challenges, such as preserving the quality of life during these extended years. *Geriatric Psychiatry,* edited by Dr. Mellow, focuses on the growing field of geriatric psychiatry, from the points of view of depression (Chapter 1, by Dr. Mellow), dementia (Chapter 2, by Dr. Weiner), psychoses (Chapter 3, by Drs. Grossberg and Desai), late-life addictions (Chapter 4, by Drs. Blow and Oslin), and public policy (Chapter 5, by Dr. Colenda and colleagues). It is clear that we are making progress in diagnosis and treatment of all of these conditions that accompany our increased longevity; it is also clear that in the future we will increasingly emphasize prevention of illness and health-promoting habits and behaviors. Because understanding motivated behavior is a main-stay of what psychiatry is all about and we still have not unraveled all of the reasons why humans do things that are bad for them, business will be brisk.

Continuing our tradition of presenting a selection of topics in each year's Review of Psychiatry Series that includes new research findings and new developments in clinical care, we look forward to Volume 23 in the Review of Psychiatry Series, which will feature brain stimulation in psychiatric treatment (edited by Sarah H. Lisanby, M.D.), developmental psychobiology (edited by B.J. Casey, Ph.D.), medical laboratory and neuropsychiatric testing (edited by Stuart C. Yudofsky, M.D., and H. Florence Kim, M.D.), and cognitive-behavioral therapy (edited by Jesse H. Wright III, M.D., Ph.D.).

Preface

Michael B. First, M.D.

In research settings, investigators routinely use structured interviews and rating scales to ensure reliable and valid assessment of diagnoses, symptoms, and outcomes. Although the need for reliable and valid measurement is no less important in clinical settings, such instruments are infrequently used by clinicians, presumably because of an underappreciation of their benefits as well as the perception that using such instruments would be too costly and time consuming. To facilitate the use of psychiatric measures in clinical practice, in 1995 the American Psychiatric Association appointed a task force to oversee the production of a handbook of psychiatric measures (American Psychiatric Association 2000). The handbook provides clinicians working in mental health or primary care settings with a compendium of the available rating scales, tests, and measures that may be useful in caring for patients with mental illnesses. For each measure described in the handbook, various information is provided, including practical issues (e.g., administration time, cost), psychometric properties (e.g., reliability and validity), and the clinical utility of the measure (e.g., in what settings the measure is useful or for what kinds of patients). However, because the mission of the handbook was to include a broad range of measures (i.e., more than 550 measures were included), little in-depth information was presented regarding the real-world issues involved in the implementation of measures in actual clinical settings. This second section of the 2003 Review of Psychiatry series, *Standardized Evaluation in Clinical Practice*, provides the reader with in-depth examination of the issues involved in using assessment tools in clinical settings. It includes five chapters, the first three focusing on the use of structured diagnostic interviews in clinical practice and the remaining two focusing on specific types of measures, namely measures for assessing suicide risk and a measure for assessing global functioning.

The central question regarding the use of structured assessments in clinical practice is immediately raised in the title of the first chapter by Monica Ramirez Basco: is there a place for research diagnostic methods in clinical settings? She correctly surmises that, to justify the use of potentially time-consuming research methodology in a busy clinical setting, it must first be demonstrated both that current diagnostic procedures are lacking and that these deficiencies might be addressed by the adoption of structured diagnostic interviews, the current gold standard for psychiatric diagnosis in research. She points out that accurate psychiatric diagnoses are clinically important to match patients to appropriate treatments, to facilitate treatment planning and risk prevention, and to improve efforts to provide psychoeducation to patients and families. Dr. Basco then reviews a number of studies to support the contentions that in a number of different settings psychiatric diagnoses are often inaccurate (e.g., Miller et al. 2001; Tiemens et al. 1999), that assessment of psychiatric comorbidity is often missed (e.g., Basco et al. 2000; King et al. 2000; Zimmerman and Mattia 1999b), that racial and cultural differences may reduce diagnostic accuracy (e.g., Flaskerud and Hu 1992; Ruiz 1995; Rumble et al. 1996), and that age biases may affect diagnostic accuracy (e.g., Class et al. 1996).

One solution to these problems in diagnostic assessment presented by the author is the implementation of structured diagnostic interviews. Basco describes and presents data on the Diagnostic Update Project (Basco et al. 2000), a collaboration between the Texas Department of Mental Health and Mental Retardation (MHMR) and the University of Texas Southwestern Medical Center at Dallas that investigated whether diagnostic accuracy could be improved by bringing research methods into the Texas MHMR system. As part of this project, one research nurse and two nurses hired from the ranks of the community mental health system were trained in administration of the Structured Clinical Interview for DSM-IV Axis I Disorders (SCID), a widely used research diagnostic assessment tool, and in making diagnoses based on interview and medical chart data. Based on the project's findings, Basco demonstrates both a significant gap between research-quality diagnostic evaluations and the results of unstructured clinical assessment practices and suggests that the gap can be bridged by utilizing trained nurses to administer research diagnostic interviews in community mental health settings. Given the limited resources typically available in such settings, Basco recommends that it might be most cost-effective to target research assessments toward groups of individuals who are most difficult to evaluate, who are most likely to be misdiagnosed, and whose misdiagnosis leads to a consumption of greater than expected amounts of treatment resources.

In the second chapter, Mark Zimmerman describes the Rhode Island Methods to Improve Diagnostic Assessment and Services (MIDAS) project, in which a comprehensive diagnostic evaluation (which includes a structured diagnostic assessment using a modified version of the SCID as well as the Structured Interview for DSM-III Personality Disorders) is given to patients in the setting of a private outpatient practice. The practical issues involved in trying to incorporate a structured assessment into a busy clinical practice are discussed, including the logistics of scheduling the evaluation (it is done in the morning of the evaluation day by a trained diagnostic rater; the results are then discussed with the treating psychiatrist before he sees the patient, usually later the same day) and concerns that the evaluation process might interfere with the development of a therapeutic alliance (which were unfounded based on an examination of dropout rates).

Zimmerman notes that because it was unlikely that comprehensive structured interviews would be incorporated into many other clinical practices, a self-administered questionnaire (called the Psychiatric Diagnostic Screening Questionnaire [PDSQ]) was developed to screen for the most common DSM-IV Axis I disorders diagnosed in outpatient settings (Zimmerman and Mattia 1999c, 2001a, 2001b). The history of the development of the PDSQ as well as reliability and validity data are presented.

In contrast to the work of Basco (in the previous chapter), which focused primarily on improvements in diagnostic accuracy, Zimmerman focuses his work on the underrecognition and underreporting of diagnostic comorbidity. Data from the MIDAS project demonstrated that the patients given a diagnosis using the modified SCID were much more likely to receive two or more diagnoses (Zimmerman and Mattia 1999b). The underrecognition of comorbidity is potentially problematic because diagnostic comorbidity predicts poorer outcome for patients with depressive and anxiety disorders, and the presence of multiple psychiatric disorders is associated with greater levels of psychosocial impairment (Grunhaus 1988; Keller et al. 1984; Noyes et al. 1990).

Zimmerman also summarizes the results from MIDAS project studies examining various other aspects of diagnostic comorbidity (e.g., comparing comorbidity rates in patients with and without a particular diagnosis [Zimmerman and Mattia 1999a]) as well as studies examining other nosologic issues that might be of interest to practitioners (e.g., whether the high rate of diagnostic comorbidity between posttraumatic stress disorder and major depressive disorder is the result of symptom overlap between the disorders [Franklin and Zimmerman 2001]). The chapter closes with a cogent discussion of whether improving diagnostic accuracy in community settings is worth the effort, given the broad spectrum of most of the currently available treatments. Although he calls for more research on whether improved diagnostic practice results in improved outcome, Zimmerman notes that awareness of comorbid conditions increases the likelihood that they will be successfully treated and that better diagnostic practice can result in greater patient satisfaction with the diagnostic assessment, an improved alliance with the treating clinician, and consequently greater compliance with treatment.

In the third chapter, Chris Lucas considers the use of structured interviews in the diagnostic assessment of children and adolescents. In contrast to the chapters by Basco and Zimmerman, which consider the use of semistructured interviews administered by clinically trained mental health care professionals, the chapter by Lucas focuses on the use of fully structured diagnostic interviews that can be administered either by lay interviewers or by computer. Lucas argues that one of the reasons why standardized diagnostic assessments are rarely part of the evaluation process in most clinical outpatient services is that they require clinical expertise that is arguably better spent on the routine complex clinical assessment that incorporates information about symptoms, context, and reactive or personality style and that is essential for treatment planning. Fully structured interviews have been developed for epidemiological research to meet a specific need for reliable measures that can be given to a large number of subjects at lower cost than can be achieved with methods that require clinicians. These cost-efficiency requirements mirror the needs of understaffed clinical providers of services for children and adolescents, making the case for the utility of fully structured interviews in clinical settings.

Lucas then describes the various versions of the Diagnostic Interview Schedule for Children (DISC), starting with the DSM-III version (DISC-1) first developed in 1984 (Costello et al. 1984) up to the current version, the DISC-IV. Data are also presented summarizing the reliability, validity, and user acceptability of the more recent versions (e.g., Schwab-Stone et al. 1996). Two recently developed versions of the DISC have particular appeal in clinical settings: the Computerized Diagnostic Interview Schedule for Children (C-DISC), in which a computer controls the diagnostic flow by presenting questions for the lay interviewer to administer to subjects, and the Voice DISC, in which the computer reads the questions aloud to the subject using a natural voice while simultaneously displaying the text on a computer monitor. The Voice DISC may provide an advantage over interviewer-administered forms of the DISC because some subjects might prefer revealing some types of very personal information to a computer rather than to a human interviewer.

In the fourth chapter, Maria Oquendo, Batsheva Halberstam, and J. John Mann discuss the utility and limitations of research instruments for a clinically crucially important purpose: the determination of suicide risk. Studies suggest that recognition and identification of imminent suicide victims by clinicians is currently poor (e.g., Isacsson et al. 1992). The chapter first presents the inherent difficulties involved in predicting risk for suicidal behavior, beginning with the lack of uniform nomenclature or classification for suicidal behavior (O'Carroll et al. 1996). The authors then explore the underlying clinical risk factors for suicide based on their proposed stress-diathesis model for suicidal behavior (Mann et al. 1999). In this model, suicidal behavior requires a trigger (stress) that interacts with an underlying vulnerability to suicidal behavior (diathesis). Clinical factors indicating a possible diathesis toward suicidality include impulsivity, a tendency for pessimism, perceiving fewer reasons for living, chronic substance abuse, chronic lack of social support, and a history of suicide attempts. The presence of one or more of these risk factors affecting the diathesis should heighten the monitoring of the patient's exposure to stressors.

Research assessments of suicide risk, although superior to clinical assessments—at least in the one study that compared the two (Malone et al. 1995)—have yet to yield an approach for determining suicide risk with good sensitivity and specificity. Nonetheless, Oquendo and colleagues note that the use of suicide scales, especially in combination, improves detection of suicidal behavior and risk for suicide and also improves the documentation of patients' suicidal behavior, ideation, intent, and hopelessness. The chapter concludes with a review of a number of available suicide scales, including the Columbia Suicide History Form, a semistructured instrument that asks about lifetime suicide attempts, method, lethality, precipitant, and surrounding circumstances (Oquendo et al. 1999); the Scale for Suicide Ideation, a reliable instrument for measuring an individual's severity of suicidal ideation (Beck et al. 1988); the Suicide Intent Scale, a 20-item scale that assesses the attempter's purpose in making an attempt, how he or she perceived the potential lethality of the attempt, and how "rescuable" the attempter thought he or she would be (Beck et al. 1974a); the Lethality Scale, assessing the degree of medical lethality or damage in a suicide attempt (Beck et al. 1975); the Hopelessness Scale, a 20-item self-report scale that measures an individual's pessimism about his or her future (Beck et al. 1974b); and the Reason for Living Inventory, which evaluates protective factors against suicidal behavior (Linehan et al. 1983).

This book concludes with a practical consideration of the organizational challenges involved in attempting to implement a structured assessment scale on a systemwide level. In the final chapter, William W. Van Stone, Kathy Henderson, Rudolf H.

Moos, Robert Rosenheck, and Mary Schohn present the issues and challenges involved in the attempt by the U.S. Department of Veterans Affairs (VA) to implement a national program of requiring the routine use of the Global Assessment of Functioning (GAF) scale in its mental health care delivery system. In 1991, in an attempt to predict hospital costs by measuring illness severity, it was mandated that psychiatric clinicians provide a GAF rating for all patients discharged from a VA psychiatric bed setting or, for those not discharged, annually at the end of each fiscal year. Despite this mandate, 80% of the GAF entries were rated as 0 (inadequate data), and only 12 of 150 hospitals were deemed fully compliant with the directive, indicating that outside incentives are needed for the success of any national program.

The GAF scale was chosen as a measurement of illness severity and functional impairment for three main reasons: it requires little time from busy clinicians who were already familiar with their patients, training was thought to be unnecessary because the scale had been part of the DSM-III-R and DSM-IV multiaxial evaluation since 1987, and the scale was designed to measure levels of both functioning and symptoms.

Software and procedures were developed to allow for the collection of GAF scores at entry into treatment and at discharge and for the transfer of GAF scores from the individual facilities to the central database in Austin, Texas. Once the software was up and running, it was still critical to obtain sufficient system compliance to have a credible database. Therefore, in 1999 the VA initiated a national performance measure (an incentive system tied in with the directors' bonuses and ratings) to get the 21 network directors and the 150 or so facility directors they supervise behind the task of ensuring that the GAF scores were obtained for all mental health patients and that they were recorded and transmitted. These efforts produced positive results: the number of patients eligible for a GAF who had a GAF score recorded in the national database gradually rose from an average (for each network) of 46% in 1998 to an average of 66% in fiscal year 2002.

The chapter then examines specific measures taken by two of the VA networks that helped improve the implementation of the GAF scale as a routine outcome measure. These included the development of training programs designed to improve the accuracy of GAF scoring and the development of a computerized performance measure monitoring system that gives the user the ability to see which patients have and have not had GAF scores completed.

The final chapter concludes with a summary of studies that analyzed the GAF data to address four important issues (Moos et al. 2000, 2002): 1) the reliability of the clinicians' GAF ratings, 2) the association between GAF ratings and other measures of patients' social and occupational functioning, 3) the association between GAF ratings and service utilization, and 4) whether GAF ratings predict treatment outcomes. The results of the analysis indicated 1) that the reliability of GAF ratings, determined by measuring clinicians' agreement with their own ratings made within an interval of no more than 7 days, was high (around 0.80); 2) that GAF ratings were somewhat associated with patients' diagnosis and symptom severity, but they were only minimally associated with patients' social and occupational functioning; 3) that GAF ratings were not closely associated with patients' receipt of services in an index episode of care as measured by the VA patient care databases; and 4) there was little if any relationship between GAF ratings and symptom or social/ occupational outcomes. The authors conclude that, although it is intuitively appealing, a brief rating of global functioning may not be able to capture changes in psychological, social, and occupational functioning that at best are only moderately interrelated.

References

American Psychiatric Association: Handbook of Clinical Measures. Washington, DC, American Psychiatric Association, 2000

Basco MR, Bostic JQ, Davies D, et al: Methods to improve diagnostic accuracy in a community mental health setting. Am J Psychiatry 157: 1599–1605, 2000

Beck A, Schuyler D, Herman J: Development of suicidal intent scales, in The Prediction of Suicide. Edited by Beck A, Resnick K, Letierri D. Bowie, MD, Charles Press, 1974a, pp 45–56

Beck AT, Weissman A, Lester D, et al: The measurement of pessimism: the hopelessness scale. J Consult Clin Psychol 42:861–865, 1974b

Beck AT, Beck R, Kovacs M: Classification of suicidal behaviors: I. Quantifying intent and medical lethality. Am J Psychiatry 132:285–287, 1975

Beck AT, Steer RA, Ranieri WF: Scale for Suicide Ideation: psychometric properties of a self-report version. J Clin Psychol 44:499–505, 1988

Class CA, Unverzagt FW, Gao S, et al: Psychiatric disorders in African American nursing home residents. Am J Psychiatry 153:677–681, 1996

Costello AJ, Edelbrock C, Dulcan MK, et al: Report on the NIMH Diagnostic Interview Schedule for Children (DISC). Washington, DC, National Institute of Mental Health, 1984

Flaskerud JH, Hu LT: Relationship of ethnicity to psychiatric diagnosis. J Nerv Ment Dis 180:296–303, 1992

Franklin CL, Zimmerman M: Posttraumatic stress disorder and major depressive disorder: investigating the role of overlapping symptoms in diagnostic comorbidity. J Nerv Ment Dis 189:548–551, 2001

Grunhaus L: Clinical and psychobiological characteristics of simultaneous panic disorder and major depression. Am J Psychiatry 145:1214–1221, 1988

Isacsson G, Boethius G, Bergman U: Low level of antidepressant prescription for people who later commit suicide: 15 years of experience from a population-based drug database in Sweden. Acta Psychiatr Scand 85:444–448, 1992

Keller MB, Klerman GL, Lavori PW, et al: Long-term outcomes of episodes of major depression. JAMA 252:788–792, 1984

King RD, Gaines LS, Lambert EW, et al: The co-occurrence of psychiatric and substance use diagnoses in adolescents in different service systems: frequency, recognition, cost, and outcomes. J Behav Health Serv Res 27:417–430, 2000

Linehan MM, Goodstein JL, Nielsen SL, et al: Reasons for staying alive when you are thinking of killing yourself: the reasons for living inventory. J Consult Clin Psychol 51:276–286, 1983

Malone KM, Szanto K, Corbitt EM, et al: Clinical assessment versus research methods in the assessment of suicidal behavior. Am J Psychiatry 152:1601–1607, 1995

Mann JJ, Waternaux C, Haas GL, et al: Towards a clinical model of suicidal behavior in psychiatric patients. Am J Psychiatry 156:181–189, 1999

Miller PR, Dasher R, Collins R, et al: Inpatient diagnostic assessments: 1. Accuracy of structured vs. unstructured interviews. Psychiatry Res 105:255–264, 2001

Moos R, McCoy L, Moos B: Global assessment of functioning (GAF) ratings: determinants and role as predictors of 1-year service use and treatment outcome. J Clin Psychol 56:449–461, 2000

Moos R, Nichol A, Moos B: Global Assessment of Functioning (GAF) ratings and the allocation and outcome of mental health care. Psychiatr Serv 53:730–737, 2002

Noyes R, Reich J, Christiansen J, et al: Outcome of panic disorder. Arch Gen Psychiatry 47:809–818, 1990

O'Carroll PW, Berman AL, Maris RW, et al: Beyond the Tower of Babel: a nomenclature for suicidology. Suicide Life Threat Behav 26:237–252, 1996

Oquendo MA, Malone KM, Ellis SP, et al: Inadequacy of antidepressant treatment of patients with major depression who are at risk for suicidal behavior. Am J Psychiatry 156:190–194, 1999

Ruiz P: Assessing, diagnosing, and treating culturally diverse individuals: a Hispanic perspective. Psychiatr Q 66:329–341, 1995

Rumble S, Swartz L, Parry C, et al: Prevalence of psychiatric morbidity in the adult population of a rural South African village. Psychol Med 26:997–1007, 1996

Schwab-Stone ME, Shaffer D, Dulcan MK, et al: Criterion validity of the NIMH Diagnostic Interview Schedule for Children (DISC-2.3). J Am Acad Child Adolesc Psychiatry 35:878–888, 1996

Tiemens BG, VonKorff M, Lin EHB: Diagnosis of depression by primary care physicians versus a structured diagnostic interview: understanding discordance. Gen Hosp Psychiatry 21:87–96, 1999

Zimmerman M, Mattia JI: Axis I diagnostic comorbidity and borderline personality disorder. Compr Psychiatry 40:245–252, 1999a

Zimmerman M, Mattia JI: Psychiatric diagnosis in clinical practice: is comorbidity being missed? Compr Psychiatry 40:182–191, 1999b

Zimmerman M, Mattia JI: The reliability and validity of a screening questionnaire for 13 DSM-IV Axis I disorders (the Psychiatric Diagnostic Screening Questionnaire) in psychiatric outpatients. J Clin Psychiatry 60:677–683, 1999c

Zimmerman M, Mattia JI: The Psychiatric Diagnostic Screening Questionnaire: development, reliability and validity. Compr Psychiatry 42:175–189, 2001a

Zimmerman M, Mattia JI: A self-report scale to help make psychiatric diagnoses: the Psychiatric Diagnostic Screening Questionnaire (PDSQ). Arch Gen Psychiatry 58:787–794, 2001b

Chapter 1

Is There a Place for Research Diagnostic Methods in Clinic Settings?

Monica Ramirez Basco, Ph.D.

The Importance of Diagnoses in Psychiatry

Clinicians differ in their views regarding the necessity and importance of psychiatric diagnoses. In the era of managed care, payment for services has become contingent on the provision of a code for reimbursable costs, and therefore the economics of mental health care has helped drive the movement toward categorical assessment of psychopathology. In many cases, the diagnosis code has no real clinical relevance in that it does not always influence interventions that are more problem or symptom focused. This is particularly true with psychotherapy or other nonpharmacological treatments.

The development of new and improved treatment strategies is contingent on the attainment of a better understanding of the biopsychosocial aspects of psychiatric illnesses. An ability to study large groups of individuals who present with similar symptoms and features of an illness allows researchers and clinicians to identify common patterns. Diagnostic classification systems aid the identification of these subgroups for which new interventions are developed and on whom they are tested. As pharmacological and nonpharmacological treatments become more refined and targeted for specific forms of mental illness, greater accuracy in diagnosis is needed so that patients can be matched to an appropriate treatment.

In many cases, knowing a patient's diagnosis allows a clinician to make predictions about his or her likely course of illness and response to treatment. This facilitates treatment planning and risk prevention efforts. When clinicians inform patients about their diagnoses, the patients can become engaged in the process of shaping their treatment, are enabled to make decisions about modifying their lifestyle to prevent relapse, can participate in discussions of long-term treatment compliance, and become more able to make realistic predictions about their future.

Problems With Psychiatric Diagnoses

Although they are essential to clinical practice, psychiatric diagnoses are often difficult to determine. As Alarcon (1995) explains, the symptoms of these disorders are typically subjective, subtle, and more intangible than the physical symptoms of general medical conditions. And unlike the diagnosis of other medical disorders, the determination of psychiatric disorders is "eminently clinical; that is, based on the personal contact between the clinician and patient" (p. 451). This introduces any number of sources of variance in the diagnostic process stemming from the patient, the clinician, and the interaction of the two, which may account for the limited accuracy of diagnostic assessments in psychiatry.

Labeling of Patients

Crowe (2000) argues that although the assignment of diagnostic labels to patients is required in most treatment settings, limiting the assessment to a categorical assignment does not do justice to the person's distress. Diagnostic labels may imply a certain degree of severity and a certain quality of life, but they cannot fully describe the individual experiences of each patient or the impact of his or her symptoms on the family, work, or social group; nor do they incorporate information about the coping resources used to offset deficits caused by the disorder.

Furthermore, the use of a categorical system for psychopathology has contributed to the common practice of referring to people as their disorders. Rather than being considered as individuals having an illness called schizophrenia, people are referred to as schizophrenics, which implies that the whole of that individual can be captured in a single label. Overgeneralization across patient types, ignorance of how psychosocial factors affect patient distress, and depersonalization and stigmatization are among the criticisms of such a diagnostic process. Unfortunately, clinicians can be as guilty as the lay public of stereotyping people with mental illness—by making assumptions about their functioning without asking questions and by viewing psychiatric patients as inferior human beings. These biases inevitably affect interactions with patients, credence given to patients' observation, and the value placed on patients' contributions to treatment plans. Voicing displeasure with the negative attitudes of clinicians is often received as evidence of pathology or as resistance to treatment. Patients' displeasure with mental health providers may be more justified than most are willing to admit.

Relying on stereotypes of mental illness can lead clinicians to jump to conclusions when only one or two symptoms are described or observed, and fail to seek out other explanations for distress. Errors of this nature are critical if they mislead the selection of treatment.

Frequency of Inaccurate or Incomplete Diagnoses

Until recent years, the accuracy of diagnoses made by primary care doctors, psychiatrists, and other mental health providers has been unquestioned. The assumption in teaching students of psychology and psychiatry has been that if adequate information were provided in the course of training along with clinical examples of psychiatric disorders, students would learn to correctly identify psychiatric cases. The gap between textbook learning and clinical application was assumed to be minimal. Because the reliability of psychiatric diagnoses is generally not systematically measured among students, drift in diagnostic accuracy goes unnoticed. The students become the teachers of the next generation, traditional teaching methods are followed, and the problem of diagnostic inaccuracy is perpetuated. To test the accuracy of diagnoses made by residents using traditional interview methods followed by consultation with an attending psychiatrist, Miller et al. (2001) compared these diagnoses to those derived by a panel of three expert diagnosticians reviewing information gathered from the Structured Clinical Interview for DSM-III-R (SCID) (Spitzer et al. 1990) and other available clinical data. Analyses showed reliability estimates of $\kappa=0.43$, which is considered only a fair level of agreement. In comparison, diagnoses derived from SCID interviews and a computer-assisted diagnostic interview (CADI) achieved reliability levels of $\kappa=0.82$ (SCID) and $\kappa=0.81$ (CADI) compared with the expert consensus diagnosis.

Problems with diagnostic accuracy are not limited to psychiatric syndromes or disorders. Even the accurate assessment of the presence or absence of a single symptom, such as delusions, can be challenging. Clinicians ranging in levels of clinical experience were asked to rate case vignettes for the presence of bizarre delusions, the presence of nondelusional abnormal ideas, or no delusions using criteria from DSM-III, DSM-III-R, and DSM-IV (American Psychiatric Association 1980, 1987, 1994; Mojtabai and Nicholson 1995). The reliabilities of the assessments were relatively low, ranging from 0.38 to 0.43. Previous experience or current contact with psychotic patients did not affect the scores, nor did the version of DSM.

In primary care settings, where patients often present with nonpsychotic mental illnesses such as anxiety and depression, the accuracy of diagnoses made by non–psychiatrically trained physicians has come under scrutiny. Kirmayer et al. (1993) investigated primary care physicians' recognition of depression and anxiety by comparing diagnoses derived from the Diagnostic Interview Schedule (DIS) (Robins et al. 1981) and the Center for Epidemiologic Studies Depression Scale (CES-D) (Radloff 1977) to documentation of mental illness in patients' medical records. Primary care physicians documented the occurrence of psychiatric distress in only 45% of the patients with high scores on the CES-D (which indicates the presence of clinically significant depression) and in only 55% of the cases identified by the DIS. When specific diagnoses were compared, only 34% of the diagnoses made by physicians and the DIS matched.

To examine the types of diagnostic errors made by primary care doctors (Tiemens et al. 1999), the accuracy, false-positive, and false-negative rates of psychiatric diagnoses rendered by primary care physicians were verified with the Composite International Diagnostic Interview—Primary Health Care Version (CIDI-PHC) (World Health Organization 1990). In a sample of 713 outpatients, the CIDI and primary care physician diagnoses agreed on the presence or absence of mental illness in nearly 75% of the sample. Agreement on the presence of depression occurred in 10% of the sample. When disagreements occurred, the majority were false negatives. Of 104 false negatives, 40 were misdiagnoses. In 27 cases the presence of a psychiatric illness was missed altogether, and in 37 cases the severity of psychiatric problems was underestimated by the primary care physician.

The problems with determination of accuracy in psychiatric diagnoses are perhaps worse for children and adolescents. Average κ reliability scores comparing structured diagnostic interviews to clinician evaluations range from 0.03 to 0.60, with averages across diagnoses within studies ranging from 0.22 to 0.31 (Jensen and Weisz 2002). Accuracy improves only modestly when structured parent interviews are obtained (Ezpeleta et al. 1997). Jensen and Weisz (2002) suggest that the amount of disagreement between structured and unstructured evaluation methods may not simply be a matter of poor reliability among raters. Instead, the diagnostic criteria developed for children may not adequately reflect their symptomatology. Before a mental illness has fully developed into a form recognizable in adults, variations in symptom presentation may occur. These variations can make it difficult for even experienced diagnosticians to identify specific disorders. Longitudinal assessment may be the valid method for assessing psychiatric and psychological phenomena in children.

In the past few decades, rigor in psychiatric research has increased as disease-specific assessment and treatment studies have required improved precision in identifying true cases of the disorders of interest. Methods to better screen for psychopathology have been developed, and more objective and thorough diagnostic procedures have followed. Although they are critical to valid research, these methods have obvious applicability to clinical service. Accurate determination of psychiatric and psychological problems would facilitate treatment selection.

To help bridge the gap between research practices and clinical services, collaborative programs throughout the United States have linked community mental health programs and university-based research programs. One such collaboration was developed between the Texas Department of Mental Health and Mental Retardation (MHMR) and the University of Texas Southwestern Medical Center at Dallas (UTSW). This research partnership began with two basic questions: 1) How accurate are the diagnoses carried by patients receiving care in the Texas MHMR system? 2) Can diagnostic accuracy be improved by bringing research methods into the clinic?

The Diagnostic Update Project (Basco et al. 2000) recruited 200 outpatients through clinician referral and self-referral to undergo a diagnostic evaluation using the SCID administered by UTSW research nurses. The information gained from the SCID was augmented by review of each patient's medical records, and a UTSW research psychiatrist or psychologist confirmed the final diagnosis of each patient after a brief interview with the patient. This final diagnosis was referred to as the "gold standard." To answer the question of whether or not the diagnoses in the patients' charts were accurate, the gold standard diagnoses rendered by the UTSW doctoral-level clinicians were compared to the most recent diagnoses documented in patients' MHMR clinic charts. The chart-based diagnoses were usually derived from an intake interview with the patient or were carried over from a prior psychiatric emergency room visit or hospitalization. Every 2 years the treating physicians updated or verified their patients' diagnoses.

The primary diagnosis documented on the patient's chart was compared to the final gold standard primary diagnosis. *Primary* was defined by prominence, severity, and duration of symptoms. A κ statistic was used to correct for diagnostic agreement that could have occurred by chance. For example, if the research psychiatrists and psychologist had arbitrarily diagnosed schizophrenia in all cases, they would have been correct in about a third of the cases just by chance, because this diagnosis is found in about 30% of all patients in the clinic. The κ statistic reflects the percentage of agreement among pairs of diagnoses relative to the total possible agreement minus chance. In this comparison the κ coefficient was 0.45. Perfect agreement would have been 1.00. No specific patterns of disagreement were found, such as mistaking schizoaffective disorder for schizophrenia. This extremely low level of agreement led to closer examination of the correspondence between the chart and gold standard diagnoses.

An accurate diagnosis is important when it helps to guide treatment selection. However, in psychiatric practice similar medication treatments might be prescribed for more than one disorder type. For example, major depressive disorder, dysthymic disorder, and depressive disorder not otherwise specified might all be treated with the same antidepressant. Patients with bipolar I and bipolar II disorders might be given a mood stabilizer as well as an antidepressant. With this principle in mind, it seemed only necessary for the chart and gold standard diagnoses to be in agreement to the extent that discrepancies would not affect the medication selection strategy. Therefore, the diagnoses of major depressive disorder, dysthymic disorder, and depressive disorder not otherwise specified were grouped together as one diagnostic category. Bipolar I, II, and cyclothymic disorders were also grouped together. Generalized anxiety disorder, obsessive-compulsive disorder, panic disorder, and social phobia were grouped under the heading of anxiety disorders, with the same assumption that the treatment selection would be similar for all the disorders in this group. Each remaining diagnosis stood alone. At this secondary level of analysis, if the chart diagnosis and the gold standard fell within the same group (e.g., bipolar I or bipolar II) they would be considered to be in agreement. Unfortunately, reducing the level of precision required for diagnostic agreement raised the κ statistic only to 0.51.

Going one step further, in a tertiary analysis all mood disorders were grouped together, all psychotic disorders with the exception of schizoaffective disorder were grouped together, and the remaining groups and individual diagnoses were the same as in the secondary analyses. This increased agreement somewhat, but with a corresponding increase in chance agreement, raising the κ statistic to only 0.52, which was still lower than acceptable. The types of discrepancies between the chart diagnoses and the gold standard were clinically significant in that they suggested different treatment strategies and different prognoses, and they would have influenced the decision to seek additional medical evaluations. These findings illustrate the gap between research-quality diagnostic evaluations and the results of unstructured clinical assessment practices and underscore the need for improved diagnostic methods in community mental health, primary care, hospital, and emergency medicine settings.

Frequency of Missed Psychiatric Comorbid Diagnoses

Using structured diagnostic interviewing supplemented by review of the medical records, Basco et al. (2000) identified 223 comorbid secondary diagnoses in a sample of 200 psychiatric outpatients, whereas clinic psychiatrists following routine diagnostic procedures documented only 41 comorbid diagnoses in this same sample of patients receiving care in a community mental health center. The most common diagnoses missed by the clinic psychiatrists were substance abuse, anxiety, and mood disorders. Similarly, in a sample of 500 adult outpatients assessed using routine clinical interviews, Zimmerman and Mattia (1999) found that one-third of the sample with a diagnosis made using the SCID met criteria for three or more DSM-IV Axis I disorders, whereas only 10% of the sample diagnosed using routine clinical interviews were found to have multiple diagnoses.

In the Fort Bragg Demonstration Project on comorbidity of substance abuse, King et al. (2000), using research-quality diagnostic interviewing methods, found 59 cases of comorbid psychiatric illness and substance abuse in a sample of 428 adolescents, whereas providers had identified only 21 of these cases. Adolescents with comorbid disorders had greater functional impairment, and their treatment was more costly overall, than adolescents without comorbid substance abuse and psychiatric symptomatology.

The detection of comorbid psychiatric disorders in general medical populations may be even more problematic because nonpsychiatric physicians tend not to be sufficiently skilled in diagnostic assessment of psychological and psychiatric problems (Lykouras et al. 1996). For example, in a sample of 68 patients with chronic fatigue syndrome (Deale and Wessely 2000), the false-positive (68%) and false-negative (35%) rates of psychiatric diagnoses were considerable. Emergency room physicians detected only 12% of the psychiatric disorders diagnosed using the Primary Care Evaluation of Mental Disorders (PRIME-MD), a standardized questionnaire and structured interview developed for use in primary care settings (Schriger et al. 2001). In a study of Finnish general practitioners, Joukamaa et al. (1995) found that physicians with postgraduate psychiatric training were more skilled at detecting psychiatric problems in their medical patients than were those doctors without psychiatric training. On the other hand, Robbins et al. (1994) found that primary care physicians who were more sympathetic to their patients' psychological distress and who were more sensitive to patients' nonverbal indicators of distress tended to be more accurate in their assessments of psychiatric symptomatology.

Although studies have highlighted the inaccuracies in diagnosis among psychiatrists, when compared with nonpsychiatric house staff, psychiatrists demonstrate superior performance in diagnostic assessment on consultation services (Margolis 1994), particularly with older patients.

Reduced Diagnostic Accuracy Due to Racial and Cultural Differences

Unlike other branches of medicine, psychiatry treats conditions whose ontology and epistemology are based on observation of behavioral manifestations of illness rather than more objective laboratory findings (Fabrega 1992). Behavior, which is generally understood by its social and cultural context, is shaped by parental attitudes, language, the symbolic value of objects and concepts, and cultural as well as local norms for socially acceptable or relevant behaviors, which differ between cultures (Alarcon 1995).

Therefore, accurate assessment of psychological and psychiatric problems requires consideration of the social and cultural context in which the behavioral indicators of distress occur. For example, in Hispanic patients, long response latencies to an examiner's query about symptoms might be interpreted as depression rather than discomfort in expressing oneself in English or distrust of the medical community (Ruiz 1995). Likewise, lack of independence from family might be viewed as pathological rather than culturally appropriate if normal family dynamics of Hispanic Americans were unfamiliar to the diagnostician. Language barriers, difficulty identifying with mental health providers, and a belief that one should handle problems on one's own can keep Hispanic Americans from seeking out psychiatric care until the symptoms are severe (Ruiz 1995). When patients are seen in their most severe state, for example, when highly agitated or displaying psychotic symptoms, overdiagnosis of schizophrenia or other psychotic disorders might occur.

Clinicians' points of reference for what is considered appropriate versus pathological behavior are influenced by their own culture and socioeconomic status. In assessing patient behavior, it is not unusual to use one's personal experiences to judge whether a particular behavior is a symptom of an underlying disorder, idiosyncratic to the individual, or consistent with local conventions (Fabrega 1994). The cultural distance between patient and clinician is a source of bias that contributes to misdiagnosis and overdiagnosis of some disorders in some racial groups.

Although psychiatric diagnostic rules such as those found in the DSM and the International Classification of Diseases have aimed at being applicable to the broadest range of individuals, there is increasing evidence that cultural and racial factors may limit the validity of these diagnostic rules in more diverse populations. For example, in a study of the prevalence of psychiatric disorders in a rural South African village (Rumble et al. 1996), standardized measures—including the Self-Reporting Questionnaire (Harding et al. 1980) and the Present State Examination (PSE) (Wing et al. 1974)—administered to a randomly selected sample of 481 adults showed an overdiagnosis of psychotic disorders. When expert diagnosticians familiar with the culture reassessed the 11 patients with a diagnosis of schizophrenia or paranoid state, the resulting diagnoses included depression, dementia, dysthymia, and anxiety disorders. One participant, with a diagnosis of schizophrenia made using the PSE, was found to have no psychiatric illness at all.

Littlewood (1992) reported similar trends in the United Kingdom, which he attributed to British definitions of normality and stereotyping of ethnic groups. In looking at data on African American males, Adebimpe's (1981) examination of racial distribution of psychiatric diagnoses showed that relative to other racial groups, African American males are also more often given a diagnosis of a psychotic disorder, particularly schizophrenia, than are other ethnic groups. The question that has been debated is whether or not these data reflect true differences by race, inaccurate diagnoses, culturally insensitive assessment tools, or racial stereotyping by clinicians.

Relying on statistical databases in which psychiatric diagnoses were derived from a variety of sources—including medical students, psychologists, emergency room physicians, and case workers—with no procedures in place to guarantee accuracy, Flaskerud and Hu (1992) found definite patterns of racial differences in diagnostic categories. African American and Asian American patients were more likely to be given diagnoses of psychosis, particularly schizophrenia, than were Caucasian and Hispanic American patients. Caucasian and Asian American patients received proportionally more diagnoses of affective disorders than did African Americans and Latinos. Using a similar database of diagnoses derived from Los Angeles County mental health records, Kim and Chun (1993) found that Asian male and female adolescents received significantly more nonpsychiatric diagnoses, such as behavior problems, than did Caucasian adolescents. Caucasian teen males were more often given diagnoses of affective disorders than were Asian teen males, whereas Asian females were more often given diagnoses of affective disorders and nonpsychiatric disorders than were Caucasian females. The investigators attest to the accuracy of the database but offer no reassurances that the diagnostic processes in this large county mental health system are reliable or valid.

When thorough and careful diagnostic methods were used in the evaluation of African American nursing home residents—including gathering collateral information from nursing home staff and performing psychiatric, physical, and neurological examinations and cognitive assessments—rates and types of psychiatric syndromes were comparable to those reported in predominantly Caucasian nursing home patient samples (Class et al. 1996). Similarly, Basco et al. (2000) found no difference in diagnostic accuracy by race when reliability in diagnosis required an exact match between clinic doctors and the research gold standard. However, when diagnoses were grouped into larger categories requiring less precision in diagnosis to achieve a match with the gold standard, the diagnoses of non-Caucasian patients were slightly more reliable ($\kappa=0.57$–0.59) than those of Caucasian patients ($\kappa=0.47$–0.49). When diagnoses determined by the SCID administered by a research nurse who supplemented evaluations with review of the medical record were compared with the research gold standard diagnosis, no differences in reliability between racial groups were detected.

Age Biases

The PRIME-MD is a well-accepted, reliable, and structured method for assessing psychiatric symptoms in primary care patients. Although clinicians in a Veterans Affairs primary care clinic were just as likely to use the PRIME-MD with older (age 65 and above) and younger (age less than 65) patients, Valenstein et al. (1998) found that older patients were less likely to receive a psychiatric diagnosis, despite high scores on the screening questionnaire, and were less likely to receive a psychiatric intervention than were younger patients. Other studies have found that when suspected in older adults (e.g., above age 50), diagnoses made by nonpsychiatric physicians are often less accurate than their diagnoses of younger adults (Margolis 1994).

With the publication of DSM-IV (American Psychiatric Association 1994) an attempt was made to improve on earlier diagnostic systems by providing information on age-related features in diagnostic categories, as well as by presenting differential diagnoses to consider when symptoms occur in older adults (Martin 1997).

As described in the study by Class et al. (1996), use of structured diagnostic interviews in a nursing home population improved reliability of assessment. The structure of interviews such as the SCID, PSE, or PRIME-MD (Spitzer et al. 1994) is intended to reduce bias, and the question-and-answer formats facilitate the evaluation of DSM criteria. However, because cultural variations were not included in versions of DSM before DSM-IV, and issues of age were included in a special section of the DSM-IV text that is separate from, rather than integrated into, the diagnostic criteria, age and race considerations were not integrated into the structures of these interviews. If the interviewer is not aware of age and racial variations in symptom presentations, errors in determining the presence or absence of symptoms can still be made despite the addition of structure and a more thorough review of symptom groups.

Assumptions Inherent in the Diagnostic Classification System

The information provided by patients is accurate.   Wiley (1998) warns us that miscommunication and even deception is inherent in the psychiatric diagnostic process. As information is provided, emphasized, and omitted selectively, the picture painted by the patient can vary. Patients' comfort with the diagnostic process can enhance the accuracy of the data collected. To avoid being misled, Wiley (1998) suggests that corroborating information be sought from medical records, interviews with family members, psychological testing, and laboratory tests. In some cases, polygraphy may enhance the diagnostic process.

   Criteria can be applied across peoples, cultures, and socioeconomic groups.   The "category fallacy" (Rogler 1993) suggests that a nosological category of psychiatric diagnosis developed in a specific culture will be relevant to all other cultures without the need to evaluate its validity in other cultural groups. It presumes consistency without consideration of local differences. However, the signs and symptoms that constitute diagnostic categories are based on a language of psychopathology developed in Europe in the mid-1800s (Fabrega 1994) and are therefore influenced by both those cultures and that era in medicine. Most diagnostic systems have been designed to be culture-free, with disorder categories supposedly representing "pure" entities that are universal. To create universal systems for classification of psychiatric disorders, socially or culturally specific problems have to be ignored. With the development of DSM-IV, the American Psychiatric Association moved toward integration of culturally specific disease entities or variants of more universally recognized psychiatric problems by providing guidelines for consideration of cultural factors in diagnosis and by including an appendix of culturally unique disorders. However, to be more useful across ethnic and cultural groups, there still remains a need to expand the DSM categories to incorporate information on cultural variations of psychiatric disorders within the diagnostic criteria (Lewis-Fernandez 1996).

Criteria applied objectively will lead to an accurate diagnosis. Various factors can influence diagnostic decisions. For example, Pini et al. (1997) found that retirement status was positively correlated with the frequency of psychiatric diagnoses made by primary care physicians in healthy control subjects, whereas severity of physical illness was positively associated with increased likelihood of a psychiatric diagnosis in patients with depression. Increased severity of psychiatric symptoms such as anxiety with comorbid depression, suicidal ideation, and early-morning worsening of mood may increase the likelihood that primary care physicians will accurately identify psychiatric illness in their patients (Karlsson et al. 2000; Pini et al. 1997). In contrast, the presence of significant somatic complaints may interfere with the recognition of psychiatric distress by primary care physicians (Kirmayer et al. 1993).

High socioeconomic status, on the other hand, may decrease detection of mental illness (Karlsson et al. 2000) or may bias diagnostic decisions. For example, in an examination of Los Angeles County mental health clinic databases, Flaskerud and Hu (1992) found that patients with lower socioeconomic status received a greater proportion of diagnoses of substance abuse and psychosis, whereas patients with higher socioeconomic status received a greater proportion of major affective disorder and other psychiatric diagnoses.

Remedies

To be useful and consistently applied, psychiatric diagnoses should be broad enough to allow for cultural and local variations of symptom presentation; precise enough to allow for maximum specificity; clear enough to decrease the likelihood of misinterpretation; and reliable enough so that when applied across settings or clinicians a given patient will receive the same diagnosis, as well as valid representations of his or her clinical phenomena (Alarcon 1995).

To accomplish these goals, the diagnostic process needs considerable improvement. Schmolke (1999) proposes that clinicians should be trained in more ethnically sensitive diagnostic processes that would include the following: 1) assessments should take into consideration the patient's quality of life; 2) patient evaluations should include wellness as well as illness factors; 3) clinicians should have an appreciation for the dynamics of the diagnostic process between clinician and patient and how these dynamics might influence patients' behaviors and the conclusions drawn; 4) clinicians should be aware of their own strengths and weaknesses, vulnerabilities, values, and personal identity; 5) optimism should be projected as a therapeutic attitude; and 6) patients' active involvement in the assessment process should be facilitated and their perspectives and understanding should be incorporated into the diagnosis

In many treatment settings, patients are not adequately involved in the diagnostic process. It is assumed that they do not know or do not want to know their diagnoses and are therefore not informed. Basco et al. (2000) found that 56% (112) of the 200 patients in a study examining diagnostic accuracy in a community mental health setting either did not know or were mistaken about their primary diagnosis. Shergill et al. (1998) also found in their sample of 126 psychiatric inpatients that 67 (53%) had not been informed of their diagnosis. Patients with schizophrenia were the least likely to have been informed. Similarly, Klein et al. (1996) found that of their sample of 48 medical inpatients referred for psychiatric consultation by their physicians, the majority (67%, 32 patients) were not told that such an evaluation was being requested, even though 81% (39 patients) indicated that they would be agreeable to receiving a psychiatric evaluation.

Wetterling and Tessmann (2000) suggest that clinicians are fearful that disclosure of diagnoses will lead to a worsening of symptoms in their patients. In a test of the validity of this concern, 255 psychiatric inpatients completed a questionnaire regarding their illness, its prognosis, and their interest in gaining information about their diagnosis. Of these patients, 88.6% wanted information about their illness and likely prognosis. About one-third of the patients were fearful of the information, but this fear did not decrease their interest in knowing more about their disorder. Sixty percent of the sample knew their diagnoses and were satisfied with the information that had been obtained. In the study by Shergill et al. (1998), most patients, when provided with diagnostic information, agreed with their doctors' diagnostic impressions. The interactive nature of structured interviews can be used to engage patients in the process. Active participation increases their interest, particularly when a clear rationale for the procedure is provided, such as using their responses to help select the best avenue of treatment. When patients are skeptical of the diagnostic process, the use of formal diagnostic instruments increases the face validity of the assessment procedure. Patients who reject the idea should be reassured that if no disorder existed, the results of the diagnostic test would be negative.

Another advantage of engaging patients in structured diagnostic interviews is that it clarifies how diagnostic decisions are derived. Reviewing the DSM diagnostic criteria, for example, illustrates to patients that a set of decision rules are available and that their diagnosis is not being made capriciously through the intuition or impressions of the clinician. If patients' trust in the evaluation procedure can be increased, their compliance with treatment regimens is likely to increase as well (Basco and Rush 1995).

Sometimes physicians fear that their patients will reject psychiatric assessments. Although this may be true during initial hospitalization for acute psychotic episodes, when patients are confused and frightened by their surroundings and the admission process (Sayre 2000), the data of Klein et al. (1996) suggest that this is more clinical lore than fact.

Szasz (1994) points out that the dynamic between patient and physician in psychiatric settings is different from any other specialty when hospital admission takes place against the will of the patient. In general medicine, patients are informed of their diagnoses and treatment options as a matter of practice, whereas psychiatric patients are prescribed treatments and are expected to comply without a substantial rationale. Receiving care unwillingly from a person or a treatment team creates resistance and resentment and decreases the likelihood that the patient will comply with the treatment regimen after hospitalization. Wetterling and Tessmann (2000) found that psychiatric inpatients in their sample who refused to cooperate in treatment regimens had not been adequately informed about their diagnoses.

Use of Structured Diagnostic Methods

Numerous studies attest to the improved accuracy in diagnostic assessment when structured methods are used instead of more traditional clinical interviews. For example, Miller (2001) developed a computer-assisted diagnostic interview (CADI) that helped evaluators to be more through and systematic in their evaluation of psychiatric symptoms. When administered to patients admitted to an inpatient psychiatric service from the emergency department, the CADI had superior reliability ($\kappa=0.75$) compared with a consensus diagnosis rendered by a panel of three diagnostic experts using more traditional interview methods ($\kappa=0.24–0.43$).

In a community mental health center serving individuals with severe and persistent mental illnesses, it was established that the working diagnoses derived using routine clinical practices were often inaccurate or incomplete compared with those rendered by research-trained doctoral-level diagnosticians (Basco et al. 2000). Most public health facilities do have access to research-trained clinicians. For structured diagnostic methods to be useful, they must be able to be administered by clinic personnel. In the Diagnostic Update Project (Basco et al. 2000), one research nurse and two nurses hired from the ranks of the community mental health system were trained in administration of the SCID and in making diagnoses based on interview and medical chart data. Comparing the diagnoses made by the nurses using the SCID with the gold standard diagnoses generated by the doctoral-level research clinicians, the reliability statistics were $\kappa=0.61$ when an exact match in diagnosis was required and $\kappa=0.64$ when similar diagnoses were grouped together. When information in patients' medical charts was incorporated with the SCID, the reliability of the diagnoses made by the nurses rose to $\kappa=0.76$ at the most precise levels of agreement and $\kappa=0.78$ when diagnoses were grouped by type (e.g., mood disorders, anxiety disorders). There were no differences in reliability between the diagnoses made by the research nurses and those made by the two nurses hired from the community mental health system. These findings suggest that the use of structured diagnostic methods can be feasible in community settings if resources are allocated to allow nurses or comparably trained individuals sufficient time to evaluate patients, preferably at the time of intake.

Supplementing structured interviews with all other available clinical data is referred to by Spitzer (1983) as the longitudinal, expert, all data (LEAD) procedure. Ideally, a patient should be observed over time to verify diagnostic impressions; evaluators should have expertise in psychiatric diagnosis; and all materials available to the clinician, including medical records and corroborating reports of family members, should be considered before a final diagnosis is rendered.

Employing decision-making algorithms, Yana et al. (1997) found that the use of structured methods for analysis of psychiatric symptoms was superior to psychiatrists' diagnostic decisions when both were based on the same information. Corty et al. (1993) demonstrated a high level of diagnostic reliability across pairs of raters using structured clinical interviews to evaluate patients with and without substance abuse disorders. Although the reliability was very good for both groups, agreement was highest among pairs of ratings for patients without substance abuse disorders.

Determining Where to Direct Efforts to Increase Diagnostic Precision

It could be argued that any person receiving psychiatric or psychological care should carry an accurate diagnosis, particularly when it guides the selection of treatment. Use of structured diagnostic interviewing methods or decision-making algorithms is initially more time consuming and costly than traditional clinical interview methods. Given the ever-present pressure of limited resources for the care of the mentally ill, community mental health clinics, health maintenance organizations, and other managed-care settings claim to be unable to afford such costly methods. Until it can be proved that an incorrect diagnosis is more costly than using systematic and structured diagnostic methods, change is unlikely to occur on a large-scale basis. In the meantime, assessment resources should be targeted toward groups of individuals who are the most difficult to evaluate, who are the most likely to receive a misdiagnosis, and whose misdiagnosis leads to consumption of greater amounts of treatment resources than would normally be expected.

Among candidates for more thorough diagnostic assessments are psychiatric patients who do not achieve symptom remission despite adequate treatment, medical patients whose distress and poor quality of life cannot be fully explained by their health problems, and individuals whose use of health care resources is well above average for their diagnostic reference group. For example, Bass et al. (1999) used hospital computer records to identify high utilizers of services in a gastroenterology outpatient clinic. Among the 50 patients identified as having had more than four visits to the hospital clinic in the prior year, 7 reported a history of childhood sexual abuse, 45 had at least one psychiatric diagnosis, and 24 had at least two. Thirty-five percent of the sample were also high utilizers of primary care clinics and other specialty clinics in the prior year.

To remedy the detection problem, is it better to screen more patients, to implement research procedures for assessment in mental health clinic settings, or to train or retrain clinicians to be more aware of psychiatric symptoms? Perhaps a combination of all three is needed. Studies suggest that screening methods would be most useful in primary care settings (Joukamaa et al. 1995; Linn and Yager 1984; Lyness et al. 1999), where prevalence rates of psychiatric illness range from 20% to 30%, with higher levels found in women and the elderly. For example, after screening 100 randomly selected primary care patients with the Hopkins Symptom Checklist–25 followed by the PSE (Wing et al. 1974), Karlsson et al. (2000) found improvement in detection rates using these structured methods (89.2% detection) over primary care physicians' rate of detection (36.9% detection).

Emergency room settings are another option. Schriger et al. (2001) found that among patients with no history of psychiatric illness who presented to the emergency department with nonspecific complaints often associated with psychiatric illness and who were willing to participate in a diagnostic interview, 42% were found to have at least one psychiatric diagnosis. Specialty medical clinics where studies have found high false-positive and false-negative rates of diagnosing psychiatric disorders (such as clinics treating patients with chronic fatigue syndrome [Deale and Wessely 2000]) or with low rates of detection such as gynecology (Bixo et al. 2001), dermatology (Aktan et al. 1998), or neurology (Lykouras et al. 1996) clinics would also be good candidates for introducing structured psychiatric interview methods.

Of course, psychiatric screening would not be useful in populations in which the incidence of severe psychological distress is low. For example, Coyne et al. (2000) found screening for psychiatric disorders unhelpful in a sample of women at high risk for breast and ovarian cancer. They used the Hopkins Symptom Checklist–25 and the SCID in a sample of 464 women. Fewer than 10% of the sample met criteria for psychiatric disorders.

It is insufficient to introduce research-quality diagnostic interviewers into medical and psychiatric settings without subsequent training of physicians in psychiatric nosology and symptom presentation. For example, Schriger et al. (2001) found that even when the PRIME-MD was used in an emergency department of a teaching hospital and the resulting diagnostic information was provided to emergency department physicians, the frequency of psychiatric diagnoses rendered by physicians (5%) was significantly less than that of diagnoses detected by the PRIME-MD (42%). Likewise, Linn and Yager (1984) found that providing primary care physicians with their patients' depression and anxiety rating scale scores did not increase the rate of detection as indicated by chart notations regarding psychiatric symptomatology.

Implementing a Structured Diagnostic System

There is considerable evidence that implementing more diligent assessment strategies for psychiatric symptoms will lead to greater diagnostic accuracy. For clinicians to accept research-based methods of assessment, however, they must be convinced that they can learn to implement the methods, that the results will be valid and reliable, and that the investment in time and resources will be worthwhile. Most psychiatrists do not have the time to conduct lengthy interviews, but they are leery of assessments conducted by other mental health professionals, including nurses and psychologists. Maintaining clinical accountability for the care of patients means that they are ultimately responsible for the accuracy of assessments, even when the assessments are conducted by ancillary staff.

First et al. (1996) developed a clinician-friendly version of the SCID for DSM-IV (Structured Clinical Interview for DSM-IV Axis I Disorders, Clinician Version [SCID-CV]). It simplifies the interview by providing an administration book with the structured questions and corresponding DSM-IV criteria and a separate score sheet for recording answers. Decision rules for determining mood and psychotic disorders are included in the score sheet. This format reduces the amount of paper used for each administration, making the method more cost effective. A numbering system that matches questions in the administration booklet with answers in the score sheet helps the interviewer keep his or her place. DSM-IV criteria are included alongside the questions intended to assess a given symptom. This allows the interviewer to immediately assess whether or not a patient's answer is sufficient to meet the criteria in question.

Numerous studies have attested to the reliability of the SCID in its various forms in patients with substance abuse problems, mood disorders, psychotic disorders, and anxiety disorders (e.g., Kranzler et al. 1995, 1997; Skre et al. 1991; Steiner et al. 1995). It is intended for use in adults over age 18 and has demonstrated reliability even in older adult populations (Segal et al. 1995). Ruskin et al. (1998) tested the reliability of the SCID when administered via videotelephones. This is particularly useful in clinics with limited access to expert diagnosticians. Thirty patients were each interviewed twice with the SCID by different clinicians. Fifteen received two face-to-face interviews and 15 received one face-to-face interview and one interview via videophone, which allowed the interviewer and the patient to see one another. Interrater reliability was high for all diagnostic categories in the face-to-face pairs and the face-to-face plus videophone pairs. Reliability ranged from $\kappa=0.73$ for major depressive disorder to $\kappa=1.0$ for panic disorder, suggesting that the SCID is both reliable and portable.

In a sample of 200 patients with severe mental illness who received care in a community mental health center (Basco et al. 2000), nurses were, on average, able to conduct interviews in 1 hour and 44 minutes (SD=32.6 minutes). To confirm the diagnoses, two research-trained psychiatrists and one research clinical psychologist conducted follow-up interviews. Interviews, which were intended to confirm or modify the diagnoses generated by the nurses using the SCID, lasted approximately 40 minutes (SD=18.8 minutes). The complexity of the patient's symptoms, the number of diagnoses, and the mental status of the patient determined the length of the interview. In this sample, most patients had multiple Axis I diagnoses.

The follow-up interview allows the licensed clinician time to review the SCID findings and ask additional questions of the patient to confirm the diagnosis and to explore other differential diagnoses. This two-step process gives the treating clinician the final say in all diagnoses, thereby allowing the clinician to maintain control over the evaluation process.

Cautions

As with any interview-based psychiatric or psychological assessment method, the interview is only as good as the interviewer. Judgments regarding the presence or absence of symptoms must be made by knowledgeable and clinically experienced individuals. It is not enough to know the procedures; interviewers must be able to recognize symptoms.

The ability to conduct a structured interview also requires adherence to the method. In the case of the SCID, all questions must be asked as they are written. In addition, the interviewer must be skilled in clarifying information, asking supporting questions, and exploring further when patients' descriptions are unclear. Sufficient pacing is also needed to complete the interview without fatiguing the patient.

Although structure improves diagnostic precision, the type of structured method selected can influence the accuracy of assessments. As part of the DSM-IV field trials, McGorry et al. (1995) compared four previously validated structured methods for diagnosing psychotic disorders. Although the same diagnostic criteria were used to derive diagnoses and the procedures were administered by expert raters, the percentage agreement among the four different diagnostic instruments ranged only from 66% to 77% without a correction for chance agreement. Although the results are significantly better than those achieved using unstructured methods, these findings demonstrate the imprecision inherent in psychiatric diagnosis even under the best circumstances.

Training Procedures

Most SCID training programs (e.g., Ventura et al. 1998) involve didactic training in psychopathology and implementation of the SCID, opportunities to observe live or taped interviews, practice in administration of the interview under direct supervision, provision of feedback and additional observation, and ongoing reliability assessments for quality control. At the University of Texas Southwestern Medical Center at Dallas, all second-year graduate students are trained in the administration of the SCID-CV. Training consists of two 8-hour workshops for didactics and practice in administration. Students practice administering the SCID at their clinical placement sites, which are supervised by a Psychiatry or Psychology faculty member. At the Intervention Research Center for Major Mental Illnesses at the University of California, Los

Angeles, trainees are provided with the SCID user's guide and audiotaped and videotaped samples of SCID interviews, which are co-rated by trainees. Trainees conduct SCID interviews, which are taped and reviewed by supervising clinicians. Using a checklist of interviewer behaviors (Ventura et al. 1998), trainees are provided with feedback not only on their diagnostic accuracy, but also on their ability to establish rapport, question patients appropriately, pace the interview, and clarify patients' responses.

Michael First, M.D., and Miriam Gibbon, M.S.W., developers of the SCID, provide training via workshops and supervision of videotapes for individuals interested in using the SCID in research or clinical settings. Information can be obtained at their Web site (http://www.scid4.org). Videotaped interviews are also available through this Web site to facilitate training.

References

Adebimpe VT: Overview: white norms and psychiatric diagnosis of black patients. Am J Psychiatry 138:279–285, 1981

Aktan S, Ozmen E, Sanli B: Psychiatric disorders in patients attending a dermatology outpatient clinic. Dermatology 197:230–234, 1998

Alarcon RD: Culture and psychiatric diagnosis. Impact on DSM-IV and ICD-10. Psychiatr Clin North Am 18:449–465, 1995

American Psychiatric Association: Diagnostic and Statistical Manual of Mental Disorders, 3rd Edition. Washington, DC, American Psychiatric Association, 1980

American Psychiatric Association: Diagnostic and Statistical Manual of Mental Disorders, 3rd Edition, Revised. Washington, DC, American Psychiatric Association, 1987

American Psychiatric Association: Diagnostic and Statistical Manual of Mental Disorders, 4th Edition. Washington, DC, American Psychiatric Association, 1994

Basco MR, Rush AJ: Compliance with pharmacotherapy in mood disorders. Psychiatr Ann 25:269–279, 1995

Basco MR, Bostic JQ, Davies D, et al: Methods to improve diagnostic accuracy in a community mental health setting. Am J Psychiatry 157:1599–1605, 2000

Bass C, Bond A, Fill D, et al: Frequent attenders without organic disease in a gastroenterology clinic. Patient characteristics and health care use. Gen Hosp Psychiatry 21:30–38, 1999

Bixo M, Sundstrom-Poromaa I, Bjorn A, et al: Patients with psychiatric disorders in gynecologic practice. Am J Obstet Gynecol 185:396–402, 2001

Class CA, Unverzagt FW, Gao S, et al: Psychiatric disorders in African American nursing home residents. Am J Psychiatry 153:677–681, 1996

Corty E, Lehman AF, Myers CP: Influence of psychoactive substance use on the reliability of psychiatric diagnosis. J Consult Clin Psychol 61:165–170, 1993

Coyne JC, Benazon NR, Gaba CG, et al: Distress and psychiatric morbidity among women from high risk breast and ovarian families. J Consult Clin Psychol 68:864–874, 2000

Crowe M: Psychiatric diagnosis: some implications for mental health nursing care. J Adv Nurs 31:583–589, 2000

Deale A, Wessely S: Diagnosis of psychiatric disorder in clinical evaluation of chronic fatigue syndrome. J R Soc Med 93:310–312, 2000

Ezpeleta L, De la Osa N, Domenech J, et al: Diagnostic agreement between clinicians and the Diagnostic Interview for Children and Adolescents—DICA-R—in an outpatient sample. J Child Psychol Psychiatry 38:431–440, 1997

Fabrega H: Diagnosis interminable: toward a culturally sensitive DSM-IV. J Nerv Ment Dis 180:5–7, 1992

Fabrega H: International systems of diagnosis in psychiatry. J Nerv Ment Dis 182:256–263, 1994

First MB, Spitzer RL, Gibbon M, et al: Structured Clinical Interview for DSM-IV Axis I Disorders, Clinician Version (SCID-CV). Washington, DC, American Psychiatric Press, 1996

Flaskerud JH, Hu LT: Relationship of ethnicity to psychiatric diagnosis. J Nerv Ment Dis 180:296–303, 1992

Harding TW, de Arango MV, Baltazar J, et al: Mental disorders in primary health care: a study of their frequency and diagnosis in four developing countries. Psychol Med 10:231–241, 1980

Jensen AL, Weisz JR: Assessing match and mismatch between practitioner-generated and standardized interview-generated diagnoses for clinic-referred children and adolescents. J Consult Clin Psychol 70:158–168, 2002

Joukamaa M, Lehtinen V, Karlsson H: The ability of general practitioners to detect mental disorders in primary health care. Acta Psychiatr Scand 9:52–56, 1995

Karlsson H, Joukamaa M, Lehtinen V: Differences between patients with identified and not identified psychiatric disorders in primary care. Acta Psychiatr Scand 102:354–358, 2000

Kim LA, Chun CA: Ethnic differences in psychiatric diagnosis among Asian American adolescents. J Nerv Ment Dis 181:612–617, 1993

King RD, Gaines LS, Lambert EW, et al: The co-occurrence of psychiatric and substance use diagnoses in adolescents in different service systems: frequency, recognition, cost, and outcomes. J Behav Health Serv Res 27:417–430, 2000

Kirmayer LJ, Robbins JM, Dworkind M, et al: Somatization and the recognition of depression and anxiety in primary care. Am J Psychiatry 150:734–741, 1993

Klein DA, Saravay SM, Pollack S: The attitudes of medical inpatients toward psychiatric consultation: a re-examination. Int J Psychiatry Med 26:287–293, 1996

Kranzler HR, Kadden RM, Burleson JA, et al: Validity of psychiatric diagnosis in patients with substance use disorders: is the interview more important than the interviewer? Compr Psychiatry 36:278–288, 1995

Kranzler HR, Tennen H, Babor TF, et al: Validity of the longitudinal, expert, all data procedure for psychiatric diagnosis in patients with psychoactive substance use disorders. Drug Alcohol Depend 45:93–104, 1997

Lewis-Fernandez R: Cultural formulation of psychiatric diagnosis. Cult Med Psychiatry 20:133–144, 1996

Linn LS, Yager J: Recognition of depression and anxiety by primary care physicians. Psychosomatics 25:593–600, 1984

Littlewood R: Psychiatric diagnosis and racial bias: empirical and interpretive approaches. Soc Sci Med 34:141–149, 1992

Lykouras L, Adrachta D, Kalfakis N, et al: GHQ-28 as an aid to detect mental disorders in neurological inpatients. Acta Psychiatr Scand 93:212–216, 1996

Lyness JM, Caine ED, King DA, et al: Psychiatric disorders in older primary care patients. J Gen Intern Med 14:249–254, 1999

Margolis RL: Nonpsychiatrist house staff frequently misdiagnose psychiatric disorders in general hospital patients. Psychosomatics 35:485–491, 1994

McGorry PD, Mihalopoulos C, Henry L, et al: Spurious precision: procedural validity of diagnostic assessment in psychotic disorders. Am J Psychiatry 152:220–223, 1995

Martin RL: Late-life psychiatric diagnosis in DSM-IV. Psychiatr Clin North Am 20:1–14, 1997

Miller PR: Inpatient diagnostic assessments: 2. Interrater reliability and outcomes of structured vs. unstructured interviews. Psychiatry Res 105:265–271, 2001

Miller PR, Dasher R, Collins R, et al: Inpatient diagnostic assessments: 1. Accuracy of structured vs. unstructured interviews. Psychiatry Res 105:255–264, 2001

Mojtabai R, Nicholson RA: Interrater reliability of ratings of delusions and bizarre delusions. Am J Psychiatry 152:1804–1806, 1995

Pini S, Berardi D, Rucci P, et al: Identification of psychiatric distress by primary care physicians. Gen Hosp Psychiatry 19:411–418, 1997

Radloff LS: The CES-D Scale: a self-report depression scale for research in the general population. Applied Psychological Measurement 140: 41–46, 1977

Robbins JM, Kirmayer LJ, Cathebras P, et al: Physician characteristics and the recognition of depression and anxiety in primary care. Med Care 32:795–812, 1994

Robins LN, Helzer JE, Croughan J, et al: The National Institute of Mental Health Diagnostic Interview Schedule: its history, characteristics, and validity. Arch Gen Psychiatry 38:381–389, 1981

Rogler LH: Culturally sensitizing psychiatric diagnosis. A framework for research. J Nerv Ment Dis 181:401–408, 1993

Ruiz P: Assessing, diagnosing, and treating culturally diverse individuals: a Hispanic perspective. Psychiatr Q 66:329–341, 1995

Rumble S, Swartz L, Parry C, et al: Prevalence of psychiatric morbidity in the adult population of a rural South African village. Psychol Med 26:997–1007, 1996

Ruskin PE, Reed S, Kumar R, et al: Reliability and acceptability of psychiatric diagnosis via telecommunication and audiovisual technology. Psychiatr Serv 49:1086–1088, 1998

Sayre J: The patient's diagnosis: explanatory models of mental illness. Qual Health Res 10:71–83, 2000

Schmolke M: Ethics in psychiatric diagnosis from a psychodynamic perspective. Psychopathology 32:152–158, 1999

Schriger DL, Gibbons PS, Lagone CA, et al: Enabling the diagnosis of occult psychiatric illness in the emergency department: a randomized, controlled trial of the computerized self-administered PRIME-MD diagnostic system. Ann Emerg Med 37:132–140, 2001

Segal DL, Kabacoff RI, Hersen M, et al: Update on the reliability of diagnosis in older psychiatric outpatients using the Structured Clinical Interview for DSM-III-R. Clin Geropsychol 1:313–321, 1995

Shergill SS, Barker D, Greenberg M: Communication of psychiatric diagnosis. Soc Psychiatry Psychiatr Epidemiol 33:32–38, 1998

Skre I, Onstad S, Torgersen S, et al: High interrater reliability for the Structured Clinical Interview for DSM-III-R Axis I (SCID-I). Acta Psychiatr Scand 84:167–173, 1991

Spitzer RL: Psychiatric diagnosis: are clinicians still necessary? Compr Psychiatry 24:399–411, 1983

Spitzer RL, Williams JBW, Gibbon M, et al: Structured Clinical Interview for DSM-III-R, Patient Edition/Non-Patient Edition (SCID-P/ SCID-NP). Washington, DC, American Psychiatric Press, 1990

Spitzer RL, Williams JB, Kroenke K, et al: Utility of a new procedure for diagnosing mental disorders in primary care. The PRIME-MD 1000 study. JAMA 272:1749–1756, 1994

Steiner J, Tebes JK, Sledge WH, et al: A comparison of the Structured Clinical Interview for DSM-III-R and clinical diagnoses. J Nerv Ment Dis 183:365–369, 1995

Szasz T: Psychiatric diagnosis, psychiatric power and psychiatric abuse. J Med Ethics 20:135–138, 1994

Tiemens BG, VonKorff M, Lin EHB: Diagnosis of depression by primary care physicians versus a structured diagnostic interview: understanding discordance. Gen Hosp Psychiatry 21:87–96, 1999

Valenstein M, Kales H, Mellow A, et al: Psychiatric diagnosis and intervention in older and younger patients in a primary care clinic: effects of a screening and diagnostic instrument. J Am Geriatr Soc 46:1499–1505, 1998

Ventura J, Liberman RP, Green MF, et al: Training and quality assurance with Structured Clinical Interviews for DSM-IV (SCID-I/P). Psychiatry Res 79:163–173, 1998

Wetterling T, Tessman G: Patient education regarding the diagnosis. Results of a survey of psychiatric patients. Psychiatr Prax 27:6–10, 2000

Wiley SD: Deception and detection in psychiatric diagnosis. Psychiatr Clin North Am 21:869–893, 1998

Wing J, Cooper J, Sartorius N: The Measurement and Classification of Psychiatric Symptoms. Cambridge, Cambridge University Press, 1974

World Health Organization: Composite International Diagnostic Interview (CIDI), Core Version 1.0. Geneva, World Health Organization, 1990

Yana K, Kitzuta H, Kawachi K: Decision support for psychiatric diagnosis based on a simple questionnaire. Methods Inf Med 36:349–351, 1997

Zimmerman M, Mattia JI: Psychiatric diagnosis in clinical practice: is comorbidity being missed? Compr Psychiatry 40:182–191, 1999

Chapter 2

Integrating the Assessment Methods of Researchers Into Routine Clinical Practice

The Rhode Island Methods to Improve Diagnostic Assessment and Services (MIDAS) Project

Mark Zimmerman, M.D.

In DSM-III (American Psychiatric Association 1980) the method of defining psychiatric disorders was changed from the prototypical descriptions used in DSM-II (American Psychiatric Association 1968) to the Washington University diagnostic approach of specifying inclusion and exclusion criteria (Feighner et al. 1972). The principal goal of this change was to improve diagnostic reliability. The early reviews of DSM-III suggested that it had succeeded in "solving" the reliability problem (Klerman et al. 1984), and up until recently few questions had been raised about the adequacy of diagnostic practice in clinical settings in the post–DSM-III era. However, during the past few years, several studies have raised concerns about the thoroughness and accuracy of diagnostic evaluations conducted by mental health professionals in routine clinical practice (Basco et al. 2000; Shear et al. 2000; Zimmerman and Mattia 1999d).

In 1980, when DSM-III was published, I was a graduate student in clinical psychology at the University of Iowa. During this time I began working in the Department of Psychiatry, which was then chaired by George Winokur (one of the coauthors of the Washington University criteria), and worked as a researcher in the department for 6 years. Working with Bill Coryell on one of the two inpatient units of Psychopathic Hospital I was trained in the administration of the Schedule for Affective Disorders and Schizophrenia (SADS) (Endicott and Spitzer 1978) and the Hamilton Rating Scale for Depression (Hamilton 1960). Working with Bruce Pfohl I helped develop the first semistructured interview to assess the DSM-III personality disorders: the Structured Interview for DSM-III Personality Disorders (SIDP) (Stangl et al. 1985). The three of us, along with Dalene Stangl, conducted a large psychobiological study of depression that included research interviews for depressive symptoms, personality disorders, family history of psychiatric disorders, life events, social support, and follow-up status (Pfohl et al. 1984; Zimmerman et al. 1986b, 1991). In another study conducted during my tenure at Iowa I administered the full SADS to a series of nonmanic psychotic patients, conducted 6- and 12-month follow-up interviews of these patients with a standardized instrument, and coordinated a family study of psychiatric disorders in which first-degree family members of patients and control subjects were administered the Diagnostic Interview Schedule and the SIDP (Coryell and Zimmerman 1987; Zimmerman and Coryell 1990). Thus, my initial experience in evaluating psychiatric patients, which lasted for 6 years, consisted almost entirely of the administration of comprehensive, standardized research interviews.

The structure and content of these interviews were imprinted, and when I began my clinical career I found that I was essentially administering the instruments. Consequently, my initial intake appointments typically lasted at least 2 hours, whereas my colleagues completed theirs in less than an hour. When I examined my colleagues' charts I noticed that they were unlikely to give patients more than one psychiatric disorder diagnosis. The low comorbidity rates found by my colleagues were clearly in contrast to the high comorbidity rates found in studies of patients based on research instruments and were lower than the rates I found in my patients. It was this observation, in the context of my research background, that was the impetus for initiating the Rhode Island Methods to Improve Diagnostic Assessment and Services (MIDAS) project, in which research assessment methods have been incorporated into routine clinical practice.

The MIDAS project consists of two major components: a structured initial diagnostic evaluation and standardized follow-up outcome ratings. An expanded version of the Structured Clinical Interview for DSM-IV (SCID) (First et al. 1995) (described below) has thus far been administered to more than 1,800 psychiatric outpatients presenting for treatment. The study is ongoing; consequently, the sample size in our more recent publications is larger than in initial papers. After the study was under way and was running smoothly, the full SIDP for DSM-IV was introduced, and more than 1,000 patients have been evaluated on DSM-IV Axis II. From the outset we assumed that comprehensive structured interviews were unlikely to be incorporated into many other clinical practices; therefore, we developed a self-administered questionnaire to screen for the most common DSM-IV Axis I disorders diagnosed in outpatient settings (Zimmerman and Mattia 1999f, 2001a, 2001b). The goal was to develop a measure with good psychometric properties that could be incorporated into routine clinical practice.

Because a wealth of data indicate that comorbidity is the rule rather than the exception, adequate outcome evaluation requires attention to comorbidity. An outcome instrument should also monitor psychosocial functioning and quality of life. Structured research interviews, administered either on a regular basis or simply as pretreatment and posttreatment end-point assessments, are too time consuming and thus too expensive for use in routine outpatient mental health settings. A major obstacle to implementing a comprehensive outcome program in routine clinical practice is the lack of a single user-friendly instrument that assesses each of these important domains of treatment outcome. Consequently, as part of the MIDAS project we developed a DSM-IV–based self-report questionnaire and clinician-rating system that can provide information to clinicians and clinics in a cost-effective manner.

To date, the focus of the publications from the MIDAS project has been on the initial assessment. Consequently, in this chapter

I focus on this aspect of our research-clinical practice integration. Readers interested in how we integrated the outcome ratings into our practice—and how this enabled us to examine such clinically important questions as the relative efficacy of switching or augmenting antidepressants in patients with treatment-refractory depression—are referred to the reports by Posternak and Zimmerman (2001) and Posternak et al. (2002).

Methods of the MIDAS Project

Patients who call our practice are offered the option of receiving a standard clinical evaluation or a more comprehensive diagnostic interview. Patients are told that the comprehensive diagnostic interview lasts half a day. Patients are asked to arrive at 8:00 A.M., are given two questionnaires to complete, and then are interviewed with the SCID, the Structured Interview for DSM-IV Personality (SIDP-IV) (Pfohl et al. 1997), and the Family History Research Diagnostic Criteria (FH-RDC) (Endicott et al. 1978). A trained diagnostic rater, currently a Ph.D.-level clinical psychologist, conducts the interviews. The patient is usually scheduled to be seen by the treating psychiatrist in the afternoon of the same day. After completing the standardized interviews, while waiting to see the psychiatrist, patients are asked to complete additional self-report scales. Sometimes, the interview with the psychiatrist is scheduled for another day, and patients are asked to bring the completed questionnaires at this time. For all evaluations, the diagnostic rater meets with the psychiatrist to summarize the findings from the structured interviews before the psychiatrist meets with the patient.

When this methodology was first proposed, my colleagues did not believe that this protocol could be successfully implemented in a clinical practice because it would interfere with the development of a therapeutic relationship with patients. Because the patient spent more time with the diagnostic rater than with the treating psychiatrist, it was suggested that it would be more difficult to develop a therapeutic alliance. To avoid jeopardizing the clinical practices of my colleagues, the first patients enrolled in the MIDAS project were limited to those who were scheduled to see me. When seeing patients for the intake evaluation I began my clinical interview by summarizing the results of the research interviews, and then I clarified areas of uncertainty and elaborated on topics that had been insufficiently covered. Even though I was provided with the information from the SCID and SIDP-IV, my evaluation typically lasted for an hour. It was my impression this method posed no threat to the development of a therapeutic alliance, and in fact it might have enhanced this alliance because it enabled me to collect developmental and psychosocial history information that otherwise I might not have had time to gather because of the time needed to evaluate current psychiatric symptoms. A comparison of dropout rates between my patients and patients seen in the rest of the practice revealed a higher retention rate among my patients, thereby further suggesting that the SCID/SIDP interview did not compromise the therapeutic alliance. As a result, the comprehensive diagnostic interviews were offered to patients being treated by all psychiatrists in the practice.

Through the years the percentage of patients presenting for treatment in our practice who were administered the SCID/SIDP varied according to the availability of diagnostic interviewers and patients' interest in receiving a more comprehensive interview. More recently, we have changed the policy in our practice and now require almost all patients to receive the comprehensive evaluation. Since the implementation of this change fewer than 10% of patients calling for an appointment decide to seek treatment elsewhere because they are unwilling to undergo such a lengthy evaluation. An important contributor to the success of the MIDAS project has been the support staff who schedule the initial evaluations and who have been educated about the benefits of comprehensive diagnostic evaluations, so this can be explained to patients calling to make an initial appointment.

Overview of Results From the MIDAS Project

Clinical Epidemiology

Community-based epidemiological studies of psychiatric disorders provide important information about the public health burden of these problems. Although the frequency of treatment seeking may be increasing (Olfson et al. 2002), epidemiological studies indicate that most patients in the community do not get treatment for psychiatric disorders. Seeking treatment is related to a number of clinical and demographic factors. Consequently, studies of the frequency and correlates of psychiatric disorders in the general population should be replicated in clinical populations to provide the practicing clinician with information that might have greater clinical utility. The gap between general-population and clinical epidemiological research might be greatest when examining disorder prevalence and diagnostic comorbidity. Obviously, one cannot extrapolate from community-based prevalence rates to clinical settings, where the disorder rates are higher. Comorbidity rates are also expected to be higher in clinical settings because help seeking may be related to comorbidity (Berkson 1946).

Most clinical epidemiological surveys have been based on unstructured clinical evaluations (Koenigsberg et al. 1985; Mezzich et al. 1989; Oldham and Skodol 1991). However, several recent studies have questioned the accuracy and thoroughness of clinical diagnostic interviews. Shear and colleagues (2000) studied diagnostic accuracy in two community mental health centers, one in urban Pittsburgh and the other in rural western Pennsylvania. They questioned whether clinicians apply DSM-IV diagnostic criteria in a rigorous manner and suggested that clinical diagnoses may not be very accurate. These researchers interviewed 164 psychiatric outpatients with the SCID after they had been evaluated clinically. More diagnoses were made on the SCID. Shear and colleagues found that more than one-third of patients received a diagnosis of adjustment disorder from the clinicians versus only 7% from the SCID interviewers. Only 13% of the patients were given a diagnosis of anxiety disorder by the clinicians, whereas more than half (53%) of the patients interviewed with the SCID received a diagnosis of a current anxiety disorder. The authors also found that half of the patients with a current primary diagnosis of major depressive disorder (MDD) on the SCID had received a diagnosis of adjustment disorder from clinicians. Shear and colleagues concluded that clinicians' diagnoses are often inaccurate and that this poses a barrier to the implementation of treatments that have been proved to be effective for specific disorders.

In another study of community mental health patients, this one conducted in Texas (Basco et al. 2000), psychiatric nurses administered the SCID to patients as a test of the utility of research diagnostic procedures in clinical practice. They found that supplementing information from the patients' charts with the information from the SCID resulted in more than five times as many comorbid conditions being diagnosed. A gold standard diagnosis, consisting of the SCID diagnosis supplemented by chart information and then confirmed by a research psychiatrist or psychologist after interviewing the patient, was made for all patients, and the level of agreement with this standard was higher for the nurse-administered SCID than for the clinical diagnoses.

Miller and colleagues (2001) compared diagnoses of 56 psychiatric inpatients evaluated with the traditional diagnostic assessment, the SCID, and a computer-assisted diagnostic evaluation. Consistent with the other studies, they found that diagnoses were missed by the unstructured clinical diagnostic evaluation compared with the computer-assisted interview. In addition, diagnoses based on the SCID and the computer-assisted interview were significantly more highly associated with a consensus diagnosis based on all sources of information than was the unstructured clinical interview.

These studies, together with the findings from the MIDAS project (described below) suggest that clinical epidemiological studies should be based on structured research evaluations. To obtain accurate disorder prevalence rates in clinical settings it may also be important to assess a broad range of pathology in contrast to a single disorder. Melartin and colleagues (2002) suggested that studies that focus on a single disorder find higher rates of that disorder compared with studies that assess several different disorders. It is possible that researchers who have expertise in the study of a particular disorder may be inclined to diagnose that disorder more frequently.

The MIDAS project is one of the first clinical epidemiological studies using structured interviews assessing a wide range of psychiatric disorders to be conducted in general clinical practice.

Among the strengths of the study are that diagnoses are based on the reliable and valid procedures used in research studies, and the patients are presenting to a community-based psychiatric outpatient practice rather than a research clinic specializing in the treatment of one or a few disorders. A limitation of the study is that it is based in a single site.

The characteristics and correlates of several DSM-IV disorders hypothesized to be underdetected by clinicians have been described in case series. One of the first reports from the MIDAS project focused on one of these disorders: body dysmorphic disorder (BDD) (Zimmerman and Mattia 1998). BDD is a distressing and impairing preoccupation with an imagined or slight defect in appearance. In a large case series of patients with BDD, Phillips and colleagues (1994) reported that the disorder was associated with significant impairment in academic, occupational, and social functioning. BDD was also associated with a risk of suicidal behavior (29% of patients had attempted suicide). Despite its associated suicidal risk and psychosocial impairment, many individuals are so humiliated or ashamed of their BDD symptoms that they keep their concerns secret even from clinicians who have been treating them for years. The underdiagnosis of BDD has been consistently described in case series and research reports (Phillips 1991; Phillips et al. 1993, 1994). There are some studies of the prevalence of BDD in psychiatric patients; however, these studies were limited to patients with selected Axis I disorders. The MIDAS project was the first to assess the presence of BDD in an unselected sample of patients presenting for treatment in an outpatient psychiatric setting.

In a sample of 500 patients interviewed with the SCID, 16 patients (3.2%) were diagnosed with BDD. BDD was the principal diagnosis for 3 patients (0.6%) and was an additional diagnosis for 13 patients (2.6%). In a separate sample of 500 patients who received a diagnosis before the SCID sample and who were evaluated with a standard, unstructured clinical interview, the prevalence of BDD was 0%. Patients with BDD received more Axis I diagnoses than the patients without BDD. Looking at the specific Axis I diagnoses, BDD patients were significantly more likely to have current diagnoses of social phobia and obsessive-compulsive disorder. The most frequent diagnosis in the BDD patients was major depressive disorder (MDD); however, BDD patients were no more likely to have MDD than were patients without BDD. The BDD patients were rated significantly lower on the Global Assessment of Functioning (American Psychiatric Association 2000) compared with the patients without BDD, indicating that their overall level of functioning was poorer. Across all patients the BDD patients were more severely depressed, despite a lack of difference in prevalence rate of MDD. The patients with BDD were not significantly more likely to have a lifetime history of suicide attempts or psychiatric hospitalization.

This study illustrated some of the power of the MIDAS project. We were able to examine the prevalence of a disorder that is rarely diagnosed in clinical practice and to demonstrate empirically that BDD is in fact underdiagnosed by clinicians. We were also able to examine the strength of association between BDD and other psychiatric disorders and the frequency of BDD in patients with these other disorders. This information is useful to clinicians who, because they have limited time to conduct diagnostic evaluations, can target higher-risk individuals for inquiry about BDD. Finally, we were able to establish that in our sample, patients with BDD, compared with patients without BDD, are more severely ill and functionally impaired but are not at greater risk for suicidal behavior.

We examined the clinical epidemiology of all Axis I disorders in a separate publication. Disorder frequency was examined in the first 400 patients interviewed with the SCID (Zimmerman and Mattia 2000). For patients with more than one disorder, the diagnoses were assigned as principal or additional according to the DSM-IV convention of whether it was the patient's stated primary reason for presenting for treatment. Table 2–1 lists the patients' DSM-IV Axis I diagnoses that were present at the time of the initial evaluation. The most frequent diagnosis was MDD, which was present in nearly half of the patients. MDD was also the most common principal diagnosis, with more than three-quarters of the depressed patients having this as their principal diagnosis. The second most common diagnosis was social phobia. In contrast to MDD—which, when present, was usually the

Table 2–1. Prevalences of current DSM-IV Axis I diagnoses in 400 psychiatry outpatients

	Total		Principal diagnosis[a]		Additional diagnosis	
	N	%	N	%	N	%
Mood disorders						
Major depression	188	47.0	147	36.8	41	10.3
Dysthymic disorder	28	7.0	4	1.0	24	6.0
Bipolar I disorder	8	2.0	7	1.8	1	0.3
Bipolar II disorder	15	3.8	13	3.3	2	0.5
Depressive disorder NOS	36	9.0	23	5.8	13	3.3
Anxiety disorders						
Panic disorder	18	4.5	3	0.8	15	3.8
Panic disorder w/agoraphobia	53	13.3	19	4.8	34	8.5
Agoraphobia w/o history of panic	6	1.5	0	0	6	1.5
Social phobia	115	28.8	4	1.0	111	27.8
Specific phobia	40	10.0	2	0.5	38	9.5
Posttraumatic stress disorder	59	14.8	19	4.8	40	10.1
Generalized anxiety disorder	34	8.5	9	2.3	25	6.3
Obsessive-compulsive disorder	34	8.5	8	2.0	26	6.6
Anxiety disorder NOS	60	15.0	15	3.8	45	11.3

Table 2–1. Prevalences of current DSM-IV Axis I diagnoses in 400 psychiatry outpatients (*continued*)

	Total		Principal diagnosis[a]		Additional diagnosis	
	N	%	N	%	N	%
Substance use disorders						
Alcohol abuse/dependence	25	6.3	5	1.3	20	5.0
Drug abuse/dependence	17	4.3	2	0.5	15	3.8
Eating disorders						
Anorexia nervosa	0	0	0	0	0	0
Bulimia nervosa	2	0.5	0	0	2	0.5
Eating disorder NOS	21	5.3	1	0.3	20	5.0
Psychotic disorders						
Schizophrenia	2	0.5	2	0.5	0	0
Schizoaffective disorder	4	1.0	4	1.0	0	0
Delusional disorder	1	0.3	0	0	1	0.3
Psychotic disorder NOS	7	1.8	2	0.5	5	1.3

Table 2–1. Prevalences of current DSM-IV Axis I diagnoses in 400 psychiatry outpatients (*continued*)

	Total		Principal diagnosis[a]		Additional diagnosis	
	N	%	N	%	N	%
Somatoform disorders						
Somatization	2	0.5	0	0	2	0.5
Hypochondriasis	5	1.3	2	0.5	3	0.8
Undifferentiated somatoform disorder	6	1.6	1	0.3	5	1.3
Pain disorder	4	1.1	1	0.3	3	0.8
Body dysmorphic disorder	10	2.6	2	0.5	8	2.1
Somatoform disorder NOS	1	0.3	0	0	1	0.3
Impulse control disorders[b]						
Intermittent explosive disorder	14	4.5	2	0.6	12	3.9
Trichotillomania	0	0	0	0	0	0
Pathological gambling	3	0.9	1	0.3	2	0.6
Kleptomania	0	0	0	0	0	0
Impulse control disorder NOS	1	0.3	0	0	1	0.3

Table 2–1. Prevalences of current DSM-IV Axis I diagnoses in 400 psychiatry outpatients (*continued*)

	Total		Principal diagnosis[a]		Additional diagnosis	
	N	%	N	%	N	%
Adjustment disorders	20	5.0	19	4.8	1	0.3
Attention deficit disorders	12	3.0	10	2.6	2	0.6

Note. NOS=not otherwise specified.

[a]The sum of all principal diagnoses does not total 400 because 6 patients received no current diagnoses, 20 patients received an Axis I or Axis II principal diagnosis not included in the table, 43 patients received an Axis I principal diagnosis in partial remission, and 4 patients received a current Axis I or Axis II diagnosis but not a principal diagnosis because their reason for presenting for treatment was unrelated to a psychiatric diagnosis.

[b]Impulse control disorders were assessed in a subset of 311 individuals out of the total sample of 400 individuals.

principal diagnosis—very few patients with social phobia had it as their principal diagnosis. The other diagnoses that were present in at least 10% of the sample were posttraumatic stress disorder (PTSD), panic disorder with agoraphobia, specific phobia, and anxiety disorder not otherwise specified. Most disorders were more frequently diagnosed as additional disorders rather than the principal disorder. Only the mood and adjustment disorders were more frequently diagnosed as the principal disorder rather than as an additional disorder.

Underrecognition of Psychiatric Comorbidity

The recognition of comorbidity has important clinical significance. Comorbidity predicts poorer outcome for patients with depressive and anxiety disorders, and the presence of multiple psychiatric disorders is associated with greater levels of psychosocial impairment (Grunhaus 1988; Keller et al. 1984; Noyes et al. 1990). In routine clinical settings, an unstructured interview is typically used to assess patients. Unstructured interviews, however, may result in missed diagnoses, with potential negative clinical consequences.

In an early report from the MIDAS project, the goal was to examine whether diagnostic comorbidity is less frequently identified through a routine clinical evaluation than with a semistructured diagnostic interview (Zimmerman and Mattia 1999d). Axis I diagnoses derived from structured and unstructured clinical interviews were compared in two groups of psychiatric outpatients seen in our practice. Five hundred patients underwent a routine unstructured clinical interview. After the evaluation of the first sample, a second sample of 500 patients was evaluated, although the individuals in the second sample were interviewed with the SCID. The two groups had similar demographic characteristics and scored similarly on symptom questionnaires

More current diagnoses were made in the SCID sample (2.3±1.4) than in the clinical sample (1.4±0.8) (t=11.6; P<0.001). Figure 2–1 shows that the majority of patients in the SCID sample (64.8%) received two or more diagnoses, compared with the minority of patients in the clinical sample (36.6%) (χ^2=79.5; P<0.001; OR=3.1; 95% CI, 2.5–4.1). The relative difference in comorbidity

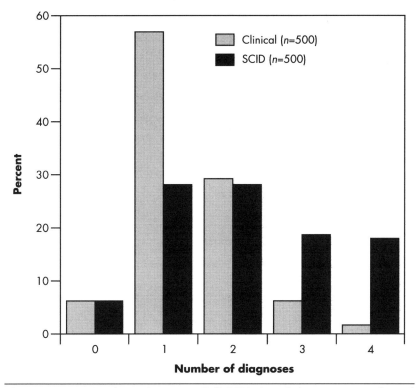

Figure 2–1. Number of current DSM-IV Axis I diagnoses in clinical and SCID samples.

Note. SCID=Structured Clinical Interview for DSM-IV.

rates between the SCID and clinical samples increased with increasing number of diagnoses: 36.0% of patients in the SCID sample had three or more diagnoses versus 7.6% in the clinical sample (χ^2=118.3; P<0.001; OR=6.3; 95% CI, 4.7–10.0); 17.6% of patients in the SCID sample had four or more diagnoses versus 1.6% in the clinical sample (χ^2=73.7; P<0.001; OR=13.1; 95% C.I., 6.3–27.4).

The data in Table 2–2 show the difference between the clinical and SCID samples in prevalence rates for specific DSM-IV Axis I disorders. Fifteen disorders were more frequently diagnosed in the SCID sample, and these differences cut across mood, anxiety, eating, somatoform, and impulse control disorder categories Chronic psychotic disorders were infrequently found in both patient series, and the SCID and clinicians diagnosed current substance use disorders with equal frequency.

Table 2–2. Frequencies of current DSM-IV Axis I disorders in clinical (N=500) and SCID (N=500) samples

	Clinical, % (n)	SCID, % (n)	Odds ratio (95% CI)	χ^2	P
Mood disorders					
Major depression	51.6 (258)	47.0 (235)	0.8 (0.6–1.1)	2.1	n.s.
Dysthymic disorder	10.8 (54)	7.4 (37)	0.7 (0.4–1.0)	3.5	n.s.
Bipolar I disorder	4.0 (20)	2.2 (11)	0.5 (0.3–1.1)	2.7	n.s.
Bipolar II disorder	0.6 (3)	3.4 (17)	5.8 (1.7–20.0)	10.0	<0.01
Depressive disorder NOS	4.2 (21)	8.0 (40)	2.0 (1.2–3.4)	6.3	<0.05
Anxiety disorders					
Panic disorder	3.4 (17)	4.6 (23)	1.4 (0.7–2.6)	0.9	n.s.
Panic disorder w/agoraphobia	9.0 (45)	14.2 (71)	1.7 (1.1–2.5)	6.6	<0.05
Agoraphobia w/o history of panic	0.2 (1)	1.2 (6)	6.1 (0.7–50.5)	+	n.s.
Social phobia	3.2 (16)	28.6 (143)	12.1 (7.1–20.7)	120.6	<0.001
Specific phobia	0.8 (4)	10.4 (52)	12.9 (4.9–34.1)	43.6	<0.001
Posttraumatic stress disorder	7.2 (36)	14.4 (72)	2.2 (1.4–3.3)	13.5	<0.001
Generalized anxiety disorder	6.2 (31)	9.6 (48)	1.6 (1.0–2.6)	4.0	<0.05
Obsessive-compulsive disorder	2.4 (12)	9.2 (46)	4.1 (2.2–7.9)	21.2	<0.001
Anxiety disorder NOS	1.4 (7)	15.4 (77)	12.8 (5.9–28.1)	63.7	<0.001
Substance use disorders					
Alcohol abuse/dependence	5.4 (27)	6.2 (31)	1.2 (0.7–2.0)	0.3	n.s.
Drug abuse/dependence	3.0 (15)	3.8 (19)	1.3 (0.6–2.5)	0.5	n.s.

Table 2–2. Frequencies of current DSM-IV Axis I disorders in clinical (*N*=500) and SCID (*N*=500) samples (*continued*)

	Clinical, % (*n*)	SCID, % (*n*)	Odds ratio (95% CI)	χ^2	*P*
Eating disorders					
Anorexia nervosa	0.2 (1)	0.0 (0)	0.3 (0.01–8.2)	+	n.s.
Bulimia nervosa	1.0 (5)	0.6 (3)	0.6 (0.1–2.5)	+	n.s.
Eating disorder NOS	0.6 (3)	6.0 (30)	10.6 (3.2–34.9)	22.8	<0.001
Psychotic disorders					
Schizophrenia	0.2 (1)	0.4 (2)	2.0 (0.2–22.2)	+	n.s.
Schizoaffective disorder	0.6 (3)	1.0 (5)	1.7 (0.4–7.0)	+	n.s.
Delusional disorder	0 (0)	0.2 (1)	3.0 (0.1–78.3)	+	n.s.
Psychotic disorder NOS	0.4 (2)	1.4 (7)	3.5 (0.7–17.1)	+	n.s.
Somatoform disorders					
Somatization disorder	0.2 (1)	0.4 (2)	2.0 (0.2–22.2)	+	n.s.
Hypochondriasis	0 (0)	1.0 (5)	11.1 (0.6–201.3)	+	=0.03
Undifferentiated somatoform disorder	0 (0)	2.2 (11)	23.5 (17.0–400.3)	11.1	<.001
Pain disorder	0 (0)	1.6 (8)	17.3 (1.0–300.3)	+	=0.004
Body dysmorphic disorder	0 (0)	3.0 (15)	32.0 (1.9–535.1)	15.2	<0.001
Somatoform disorder NOS	0 (0)	0.2 (1)	3.0 (0.1–78.3)	+	n.s.

Table 2–2. Frequencies of current DSM-IV Axis I disorders in clinical ($N=500$) and SCID ($N=500$) samples *(continued)*

	Clinical, % (*n*)	SCID, % (*n*)	Odds ratio (95% CI)	χ^2	*P*
Impulse control disorders[a]					
Intermittent explosive disorder	0.6 (3)	3.4 (14)	5.9 (1.7–20.6)	9.8	<0.01
Trichotillomania	0 (0)	0.2 (1)	3.7 (0.1–90.4)	†	n.s.
Pathological gambling	0 (0)	0.5 (2)	6.1 (0.3–128.4)	†	n.s.
Kleptomania	0 (0)	0 (0)	—	—	—
Impulse control disorder NOS	0 (0)	0.2 (1)	3.7 (0.1–90.4)	†	n.s.
Adjustment disorders	9.6 (48)	5.0 (25)	0.5 (0.3–0.8)	7.8	<0.01
Attention deficit disorders	2.6 (13)	3.4 (17)	1.3 (0.6–2.7)	0.5	n.s.

Note. SCID=Structured Clinical Interview for DSM-IV; CI=confidence interval; NOS=not otherwise specified; n.s.=not significant.
[a]In the SCID group, impulse control disorders were assessed in a subset of 409 individuals out of the full sample of 500 individuals.
†Fisher's exact test.

There are several alternative explanations for the lower co-morbidity rates in the clinical sample compared with the SCID sample. First, it is possible that the difference in comorbidity rates reflects true sample differences, and the clinical sample was a less severely ill group. Although it is not possible to rule out this explanation, the similarity in the two samples' demographic profile and scores on self-administered symptom severity scales makes it less likely that the diagnostic differences between the samples reflects a real intersample difference in level of pathology.

Second, it is possible that the lower comorbidity rates in the clinical sample are the result of clinicians' deliberate underdocumentation of psychopathology. If clinicians censor from their records diagnostic information that patients are most embarrassed, ashamed, or stigmatized by, then it would be inappropriate to conclude that comorbidity was not being detected. However, post hoc conversations with the clinicians in the practice indicated that they did not deliberately omit diagnostic information from the patients' charts.

Third, underdiagnosis may be a local rather than a widespread problem. Perhaps the clinicians in our practice are poor diagnosticians who failed to detect comorbidity. Although it is not possible to rule out this possibility, the clinical comorbidity rate found in the present study is higher than the 17%–26% rates found in three other reports of comorbidity based on clinical evaluations (Loranger 1990; Mezzich et al. 1989; Stangler and Printz 1979). Thus, it does not appear that the psychiatrists in this study were more likely than other psychiatrists to underrecognize diagnostic comorbidity.

Fourth, perhaps the problem is not with clinician underdiagnosis but with overdiagnosis by semistructured research interviews. Interviews such as the SCID are viewed as diagnostic gold standards, but it is possible that they are too sensitive and result in false-positive diagnoses. Or perhaps we were biased to overdiagnose. Inconsistent with this is anecdotal information that when the results of the SCID evaluations were presented to the clinicians, the clinicians noted more diagnoses in the patients' clinical charts. Because clinicians confirmed the SCID diagnoses and recorded more diagnoses in their patients' charts compared with when they conducted unstructured clinical evaluations, it is less likely that diagnostic bias accounts for the findings. In a report of the impact of research interviews on clinicians' diagnostic practice, we focused on the diagnosis of borderline personality disorder (Zimmerman and Mattia 1999b). We hypothesized that the diagnosis of borderline personality disorder during the initial evaluation is influenced by the amount of information clinicians have available to them at the interview, and if clinicians are provided with information indicative of a diagnosis of borderline personality disorder then the diagnosis will be made. Consistent with this, we found that the frequency of borderline personality disorder diagnoses assigned by clinicians (0.4%) increased more than 20-fold when the information from the SIDP-IV was presented to the clinicians before their evaluation (9.2%) ($\chi^2=31.97$; 1 df; $P<0.001$).

Studies of Diagnostic Comorbidity

The large size of the MIDAS project sample, together with the extensiveness of the assessment protocol, offer many opportunities to examine questions of diagnostic comorbidity. Three of these analyses are summarized below.

How often do depressed patients have at least one other current DSM-IV Axis I disorder at the time of presentation? To our surprise this question has not received much research attention. At the time we wrote our article on this topic we were aware of only one other published study of the frequency of a wide range of Axis I disorders in depressed outpatients (Sanderson et al. 1990). (One month before the publication of our study a second study was published [Melartin et al. 2002]). The question about the frequency of comorbidity seems straightforward; however, when addressing the question it became apparent that the answer is influenced by the breadth of the diagnostic assessment (Zimmerman et al. 2002a). We examined the impact of two factors related to the breadth of assessment: the range of disorders covered and the assessment of subthreshold conditions. Because our diagnostic evaluation used an expanded version of the SCID, we could compare the comorbidity rate based on the range of disorders typically covered by the SCID with the rate based on a more complete evaluation of Axis I disorders. Subthreshold conditions (often categorized as not otherwise specified) have rarely been described in studies of diagnostic comorbidity. We found that many depressed patients presenting for treatment had clinically significant symptoms of a nondepressive disorder that never met full diagnostic criteria, therefore we considered it important to describe this phenomenon to obtain a better appreciation of the number of current comorbid conditions in depressed patients. Current subthreshold disorders also include conditions that had met full criteria in the past but at the time of presentation had incompletely improved. Therefore, we also examined the frequency of disorders that are in partial remission at the time of presentation. Table 2–3 summarizes the findings on the impact of the breadth of assessment on comorbidity rates in patients with MDD. One finding that is clear from this table is that the majority of depressed patients have another Axis I disorder at the time of their presentation for treatment.

Another type of comorbidity study conducted in the MIDAS project was the comparison of comorbidity rates in patients with and without a particular diagnosis (Zimmerman and Mattia 1999a). This approach was taken in our study of comorbidity and borderline personality disorder. The patients with borderline personality disorder were given significantly more current DSM-IV Axis I disorder diagnoses (3.4 ± 1.5 versus 2.0 ± 1.4; $t=7.42$; $P<0.001$). Figure 2–2 shows the distribution of current diagnoses in the patients with and without borderline personality disorder. The patients with borderline personality disorder were twice as likely to have received three or more current DSM-IV disorder diagnoses (69.5% versus 31.1%; $\chi^2=32.0$; $P<0.001$) and were four times as likely to have been diagnosed with four or more disorders (47.5% versus 13.7%; $\chi^2=38.0$; $P<0.001$). Looking at the specific disorders, the patients with borderline personality disorder were more frequently diagnosed with MDD, bipolar I and bipolar II disorders, panic disorder with agoraphobia, social and specific phobia, PTSD, obsessive-compulsive disorder, eating disorder not otherwise specified, and any somatoform disorder. The extent of comorbidity highlights the importance of conducting thorough evaluations of Axis I pathology in patients with

Table 2–3. Current and lifetime DSM-IV Axis I comorbidity rates in 479 depressed outpatients as a function of the breadth of the diagnostic assessment

	Total		1 or more disorders		2 or more disorders	
	Mean	SD	%	n	%	n
Current diagnosis						
Dysthymic, anxiety, substance, somatoform, and eating disorders	1.25	1.30	63.0	302	35.5	170
All of the above plus impulse control disorders	1.29	1.34	64.1	307	36.7	176
All of the above plus nicotine dependence	1.56	1.45	72.2	346	43.2	207
All of the above plus partial remission	1.72	1.54	73.9	354	47.8	229
All of the above plus NOS disorders	1.97	1.63	79.3	380	53.6	257
Lifetime diagnosis						
Dysthymic, anxiety, substance, somatoform, and eating disorders	2.03	1.68	78.9	378	56.8	272
All of the above plus impulse control disorders	2.12	1.73	80.0	383	59.1	283
All of the above plus nicotine dependence	2.50	1.88	85.4	409	65.1	312
All of the above plus NOS disorders	2.81	1.94	88.9	426	71.6	343

Note. NOS=not otherwise specified.

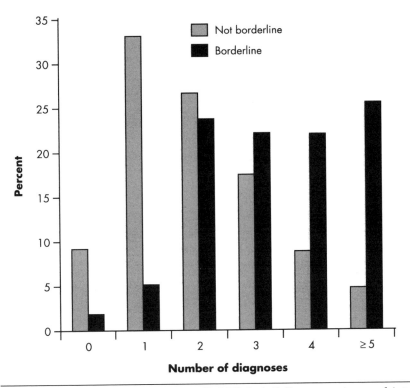

Figure 2–2. Number of current DSM-IV Axis I diagnoses in psychiatric outpatients with and without borderline personality disorder.

borderline personality disorder to avoid overlooking syndromes that are potentially responsive to treatment.

In a third type of comorbidity study conducted in the MIDAS project we examined the association between two disorders. Many studies had established that a large percentage of patients with PTSD have MDD (Deering et al. 1996; Green et al. 1989; Kessler et al. 1995; Sierles et al. 1983). Other studies have found that patients with PTSD or a history of childhood trauma have an increased rate of psychotic symptoms (Butler et al. 1996; Pribor and Dinwiddie 1992; Roszell et al. 1991). Consequently, we examined the relationship between psychotic subtyping of MDD and the presence of PTSD (Zimmerman and Mattia 1999e). Compared with patients with nonpsychotic depression, the patients with psychotic depression were nearly four times more likely to have current PTSD (15.7% versus 57.9%) (Fisher's exact $P=0.0001$). It was hypothesized that the poorer longitudinal course of psychotic depression compared with nonpsychotic depression may be due to the underrecognition of PTSD in psychotically depressed patients.

A Consumer's Perspective of the Relevance of Detecting Comorbid Conditions

Although information regarding diagnostic comorbidity can provide prognostic predictive value, such information may not be immediately useful if patients have minimal interest or willingness for treatment directed toward the comorbid conditions that are not the primary reason for seeking treatment.

As part of our modification of the SCID, for all current disorders patients are asked if the symptoms of each diagnosed disorder were a reason (or among the reasons) for seeking treatment (Zimmerman and Mattia 2000). Nearly all patients wanted treatment for their MDD, and more than 85% of patients with panic disorder, PTSD, and generalized anxiety disorder (GAD) indicated that the symptoms of these disorders were a reason for seeking treatment. Between one-half to two-thirds of patients with social phobia, obsessive-compulsive disorder, intermittent explosive disorder, BDD, and substance use disorders reported that the symptoms of these disorders were a reason for seeking treatment. Only 30% of individuals with specific phobia indicated that their phobic fears were a reason for seeking treatment. Summing across the entire sample, more than 900 diagnoses were made. Of the 505 diagnoses that were not the principal reason for seeking treatment, patients still indicated that 60% of these additional disorders were among the reasons they had sought treatment, although there were considerable differences among the classes of disorders regarding desire for treatment.

Clinical Need for a Diagnostic Screening Instrument

A complete psychiatric evaluation covering all the major domains of Axis I psychopathology must be sufficiently broad-based to include questions about the symptoms of many disorders. Because thoroughness is time consuming, it is incompatible with cost containment—the major impetus behind recent changes in the delivery of mental health care services. Insurance company strictures are resulting in briefer diagnostic interviews in ambulatory mental health settings, and concomitantly clinicians are increasingly required to complete their intake evaluations within an hour. One of the early goals of the MIDAS project was to develop a diagnosis-oriented tool that would help time-constrained clinicians use their time more efficiently and maintain or improve their level of diagnostic accuracy.

A self-report questionnaire is an inexpensive method of collecting reliable and valid clinical information. Questionnaires are commonly used by physicians in all branches of medicine to collect medical histories before a patient's initial evaluation. Questionnaires have long been used in the mental health field to evaluate personality constructs, mood, psychosocial functioning, etc. During the past 10 years some questionnaires have been designed to screen for, or "diagnose," single DSM-III/DSM-III-R (American Psychiatric Association 1987) Axis I disorders such as MDD, PTSD, and bulimia nervosa (Foa et al. 1993; Thelen et al. 1991; Zimmerman et al. 1986a). Although several questionnaires have been developed to assess all of the DSM-III/DSM-III-R Axis II personality disorders (e.g., Hyler et al. 1988; Millon 1994), at the time we began the MIDAS project no scales had been developed to screen efficiently for a broad range of DSM-IV Axis I disorders in psychiatric outpatients.

Of course, brief self-report questionnaires cannot substitute for clinical evaluations and cannot render definitive diagnoses. Therefore, the questionnaire we constructed is referred to as a screening rather than a diagnostic instrument. It is intended for use by practicing clinicians as a guide to symptom domains requiring more or less focus during the clinical interview. And although a questionnaire cannot diagnose a psychiatric disorder per se, it should be emphasized that the level of agreement between a questionnaire and a diagnostic interview can be as high as the test-retest reliability of the diagnostic interview itself (Zimmerman and Coryell 1988).

Initial Development of the Psychiatric Diagnostic Screening Questionnaire

The Psychiatric Diagnostic Screening Questionnaire (PDSQ) is a self-report scale designed to screen for the most common DSM-IV Axis I disorders encountered in outpatient mental health settings (Zimmerman and Mattia 1999f, 2001a, 2001b). Five research and clinical influences of the past two decades contributed to the development of the PDSQ. First, the publication of specific inclusion criteria to make psychiatric diagnoses, complemented by the development of standardized interviews to reliably assess the criteria, set the stage for the construction of other types of instruments such as self-administered questionnaires to screen for or make provisional psychiatric diagnoses. Research diagnostic interviews such as the SADS, the Diagnostic Interview Schedule, and the SCID have been accepted as diagnostic standards, albeit imperfect ones, to which the diagnostic performance of other tests (be they biological or self-report) can be compared.

Second, after the publication of specific inclusion and exclusion criteria to make psychiatric diagnoses, self-report questionnaires were developed to "diagnose" individual DSM disorders. One of the first such measures was constructed in the early 1980s by Zimmerman et al. (1986a), who developed the Inventory to Diagnose Depression (IDD) to evaluate the DSM-III criteria for MDD. The studies by Zimmerman and colleagues demonstrated that the level of agreement between a self-report scale and a research diagnostic interview for the diagnosis of major depression was as high as the test-retest reliability of the diagnostic interview. Moreover, their research indicated that a self-report scale such as the IDD could perform well in both patient and nonpatient community samples (Zimmerman and Coryell 1988, 1994; Zimmerman et al. 1986a). During the past 15 years their initial work on the IDD was replicated by other research groups (Kuhner and Veiel 1993), and other questionnaires have been designed to assess the criteria of different DSM Axis I disorders (Foa et al. 1993; Thelen et al. 1996).

The third influence on our decision to develop a broad-based questionnaire that assessed several Axis I disorders was the increasing research and discussion of diagnostic comorbidity. During the nearly two decades after the publication of DSM-III a large body of literature had accumulated documenting the high degree of diagnostic comorbidity among the DSM disorders (Maser and Cloninger 1990). High rates of diagnostic comorbidity may well be an artifact of the nomenclature; nonetheless, the clinical and research significance of comorbidity has been increasingly discussed (Sabshin 1991).

Fourth, as suggested above, there has been accumulating evidence that diagnostic comorbidity is underrecognized in routine clinical practice. Comorbidity rates in patients whose diagnoses are made by clinicians in the routine clinical setting are one-half to one-third the comorbidity rates reported in studies using standardized research diagnostic interviews (Zimmerman and Mattia 1999d).

And finally, the changing health care delivery system has put an increasing premium on efficiency at the expense of conducting a thorough, time-consuming diagnostic anamnesis. Underrecognition of diagnostic comorbidity may therefore be more likely when clinicians' time to conduct diagnostic evaluations is reduced.

This confluence of factors—specification of diagnostic criteria, acceptance of standardized interview–derived diagnoses as a diagnostic standard, demonstration of high rates of diagnostic comorbidity, underrecognition of comorbidity in routine clinical practice, and time pressure constraints to improve clinical efficiency—was the impetus for the development of the PDSQ. Our goal was to develop a clinically useful instrument that was brief enough to be completed by patients in a timely manner before their initial diagnostic evaluation, yet comprehensive enough to cover the most common disorders for which individuals seek treatment. Also, the scoring and organization of the measure should be straightforward enough so that a clinician, or office worker, can rapidly review and score the scale and obtain clinically meaningful information.

The PDSQ has undergone several rounds of study involving more than 3,000 primary care and psychiatric outpatients. After each large validation study the scale was revised based on a psychometric analysis of the subscales and items. The final version of the PDSQ consists of 126 questions assessing the symptoms of 13 DSM-IV disorders in five areas: eating disorders (bulimia/binge eating disorder), mood disorders (MDD), anxiety disorders (panic disorder, agoraphobia, PTSD, obsessive-compulsive disorder, GAD, and social phobia), substance use disorders (alcohol abuse/dependence, drug abuse/dependence), and somatoform disorders (somatization disorder, hypochondriasis). In addition, there is a six-item psychosis screen. The disorders chosen for coverage were selected because they are the most prevalent in epidemiological surveys of the community (Kessler et al. 1994; Robins et al. 1991) and are the most frequently reported in large clinical samples (Koenigsberg et al. 1985; Mezzich et al. 1989; Zimmerman and Mattia 1999d). Two subscales, mania and anorexia, were dropped after extensive investigation due to poor psychometric performance.

In determining the length of the PDSQ subscales we tried to balance the desire to keep the scale brief (so that it would be feasible to incorporate it into routine clinical practice) with the desire to make the scale comprehensive so that most or all diagnostic criteria of the included disorders were assessed. Because longer scales tend to have better psychometric properties, we decided that each subscale should have a minimum of five items. The major depression subscale, with 22 items, is the longest PDSQ subscale because it assesses each of the nine DSM-IV symptom criteria and includes a separate question for each element of the compound depression criteria (e.g., the DSM-IV sleep disturbance criterion is assessed with separate questions for both increased and decreased sleep). The reason for including this level of detail was the potential treatment implications of the presence of vegetative and reverse vegetative symptoms of depression. The numbers of items on the other PDSQ subscales are as follows: PTSD, 15; bulimia/binge-eating disorder, 10; obsessive-compulsive disorder, 8; panic disorder, 8; psychosis, 6; agoraphobia, 11; social phobia, 15; alcohol abuse/dependence, 6; drug abuse/dependence, 6; GAD, 10; somatization, 5; and hypochondriasis, 5.

In the validity study of the final version of the PDSQ, 994 psychiatric outpatients completed the scale. The 13 PDSQ subscales demonstrated good to excellent levels of internal consistency. Cronbach's α was greater than 0.80 for 12 of the 13 subscales, and the mean of the α coefficients was 0.86. Test-retest reliability was calculated for the 185 subjects who completed the PDSQ two times in less than a week. Test-retest reliability coefficients were greater than 0.80 for 9 subscales, and the mean of the test-retest correlation coefficients was 0.83. The convergent and discriminant validity of the PDSQ subscales was determined by comparing the correlation between each PDSQ subscale and other self-report measures of the same construct versus different constructs (Campbell and Fiske 1959). Three hundred sixty-one patients completed a package of questionnaires at home less than a week after completing the PDSQ. The booklet included measures of symptoms related to each of the PDSQ symptom domains (Beck et al. 1979, 1988; Foa et al. 1993; Garner et al. 1983; Hodgson and Rachman 1977; Kellner 1985; Leary 1983; Marks and Mathews 1979; Meyer et al. 1990; Othmer and DeSouza 1985; Pilowsky 1967; Selzer 1971; Shugar et al. 1992; Skinner 1982; Swartz et al. 1986). Every PDSQ subscale was more highly correlated with the concordant validity scale assessing the same symptom domain versus other symptom domains. Across all subscales, the mean correlation between the PDSQ subscales and their respective validity scales was 0.66, whereas the mean correlation between PDSQ subscales and measures of other symptom domains was 0.25. Finally, for each of the disorders assessed by the PDSQ, the mean diagnosis-specific subscale score in patients with and without that DSM-IV diagnosis were compared. For every PDSQ subscale, scores were significantly higher for patients with, versus without, the corresponding diagnosis.

Diagnostic Performance of the PDSQ

The diagnostic performance of a scale is usually evaluated by examining the scale's sensitivity and specificity across a range of cutoff scores. *Sensitivity* refers to a test's ability to correctly identify individuals with the disorder, whereas *specificity* refers to a test's ability to identify non-ill persons. Sensitivity and specificity provide useful psychometric information about a test; however, the clinically more meaningful conditional probabilities are positive and negative predictive values. These values indicate the probability that individuals are ill or non-ill given that they have been identified by the test as being ill or non-ill. Accordingly, *positive predictive value* is the percentage of individuals classified ill by the test who are truly ill, whereas *negative predictive value* is the percentage of individuals classified as not ill by the test who truly are not ill.

Sensitivity, specificity, and positive and negative predictive values are not invariant properties of a test—they are a function of the cutoff point used to distinguish cases from noncases. Depending on the instrument's purpose, cutoff scores might be selected to optimize the sensitivity or the specificity of the scale (Hsiao et al. 1989; Mossman and Somoza 1989). In our report of the diagnostic performance of the PDSQ subscales we examined the diagnostic statistics across the range of cutoff scores and determined the average specificity and positive and negative predictive values across the PDSQ subscales when sensitivity was 80%, 85%, and 90%.

We examined the diagnostic performance of the PDSQ in 630 psychiatric outpatients interviewed with the SCID. The diagnostic properties of the PDSQ subscales varied in a predictable manner according to the cutoff score: as the threshold increased, sensitivity decreased and specificity increased. At the respective cutoff scores resulting in a sensitivity of 80%, subscale specificities ranged from a high of 91% for the bulimia and drug abuse/dependence subscales to a low of 58% for the somatization subscale. When subscale sensitivity was 80%, the mean specificity across all subscales was 78%; when subscale sensitivity was 85%, mean specificity was 73%; and when subscale sensitivity was 90%, mean specificity was 66%. When subscale sensitivity was 80%, the mean positive predictive value across the subscales was 32% and the mean negative predictive value was 95%; when subscale sensitivity was 85%, mean positive predictive value was 31% and mean negative predictive value was 96%; when subscale sensitivity was 90%, mean positive predictive value was 30% and mean negative predictive value was 97%.

The threshold chosen for case identification will vary according to the desired use of the measure. If the goal is to ensure detection of all cases, then the threshold should be set low to increase diagnostic sensitivity (at a cost of more false-positive diagnoses and hence lower specificity). On the other hand if the goal is to identify a relatively homogeneous group with few false positives, then the user should choose a higher cutoff score with consequent improved specificity (but lower sensitivity).

The PDSQ was intended as a diagnostic aid to be used in clinical practice to facilitate the efficiency of conducting the initial diagnostic evaluation. Consequently, we recommended that a cutoff resulting in diagnostic sensitivity of 90% be chosen when using the scale in clinical practice. From a clinical perspective it is most important that the diagnostic aid have good sensitivity and corresponding high negative predictive value. With high negative predictive value the clinician can be confident that when the test indicates that the disorder is not present there is little need to inquire about that disorder's symptoms. False-positive diagnoses are less of a problem for a screening questionnaire because their major cost is the time a clinician takes to determine that the disorder is not present. Presumably this is time the clinician would have nonetheless spent for the same purpose. Based on the cutoffs resulting in a sensitivity of 90%, the mean negative predictive value of the PDSQ subscales was 97% and the false-positive rate was 34%.

We developed the PDSQ to aid clinicians in making psychiatric diagnoses. It is common in medical practices to have patients complete some initial paperwork that is reviewed before the initial visit. We recommend that the PDSQ be used in a similar way. That is, the responses to the scale should be reviewed before the face-to-face encounter, and the information thus obtained should make it less likely that areas of psychopathology are overlooked. Of course, a thorough diagnostic interview is the diagnostic standard of care. There are no special questions on the PDSQ that allow it to detect psychopathology that otherwise would go undetected during a clinical evaluation. However, clinicians often do not have the time to be as comprehensive as they would like. It is our hope that the PDSQ can improve the efficiency of the diagnostic evaluation by guiding clinicians toward symptom areas that require more versus less assessment. In a separate report we described how the PDSQ validly detected PTSD in patients who were not diagnosed with PTSD by their treating clinicians (Zimmerman and Mattia 1999c).

Examination of Nosologic Issues

In the MIDAS project we made several modifications to the SCID to permit examination of nosologic issues that might be of interest to practitioners. For example, we suspended the DSM-IV hierarchy between substance dependence and abuse and assessed abuse in patients with substance dependence. This enables clinicians to determine how often patients have substance dependence without abuse and whether patients with both dependence and abuse differ from patients with dependence but not abuse.

We were interested in whether the SCID screening questions for some disorders captured all individuals with the disorder. For social phobia, regardless of how individuals responded to the SCID screening probe about anxiety related to public speaking or eating in front of others, they were also asked if they felt more fearful, anxious, or nervous than most people in 15 different social situations. For PTSD, a negative response to the screening question is followed up by questions about 12 specific traumatic events. We added items to the depression section that are not DSM-IV diagnostic criteria to examine the validity of different methods of diagnosing MDD. We assessed all symptoms of MDD and PTSD without skipping out after the screening questions to examine the diagnostic psychometric properties of these criteria sets. During the first year of the MIDAS project we had observed that many depressed patients had high levels of chronic anxiety characterized by excessive worrying and other features of GAD, but these individuals were not diagnosed with GAD according to DSM-IV because the symptoms occurred only during the course of a chronic mood disorder. To study the validity of the DSM-IV hierarchical relationship between GAD and mood disorders we changed our diagnostic procedure and made a diagnosis of modified GAD in patients who met all GAD criteria except for the exclusion criterion.

Some of these questions have already been examined. For example, we examined the performance of the SCID's screening question for PTSD and found that although the SCID screening question had a sensitivity of about 80% for detecting a lifetime history of trauma, its sensitivity was greater than 95% for detecting PTSD (Franklin et al., in press). To study the validity of the DSM-IV hierarchical relationship between GAD and mood disorders we made a diagnosis of modified GAD in patients with MDD who met all GAD criteria except for the exclusion criterion. In our analyses we compared three nonoverlapping groups of patients: 1) patients with DSM-IV MDD and GAD; 2) depressed patients with modified GAD; and 3) MDD patients without GAD (Zimmerman and Chelminski, in press). Compared with depressed patients without GAD, depressed patients with DSM-IV GAD and modified GAD had higher levels of suicidal ideation; poorer social functioning; greater frequency of other anxiety disorders, eating disorders, and somatoform disorders; higher scores on most PDSQ subscales; greater level of pathological worry; and higher morbid risk for GAD in first-degree family members. The two GAD groups did not differ from each other. These findings question the validity of the DSM-IV hierarchical relationship between MDD and GAD and suggest that the exclusion criterion should be eliminated.

In another report, we examined whether the high rate of diagnostic comorbidity between PTSD and MDD is the result of symptom overlap (contaminated symptoms) between the disorders (Franklin and Zimmerman 2001). PTSD symptoms were subdivided into two groups: the contaminated symptoms (anhedonia, concentration and sleep problems) and the 14 symptoms that are unique to PTSD. It was speculated that if the contaminated symptoms are responsible for the comorbidity, then they will show less specificity than the unique symptoms, will be less highly correlated with a PTSD symptom total count, and will be more frequently endorsed in PTSD patients with than without MDD. None of the hypotheses were supported, thereby suggesting that the comorbidity between PTSD and MDD is not an artifact of symptom overlap.

Generalizability of Treatment Research

During the past few years there have been increasing concerns about the generalizability of the results of tightly controlled efficacy trials to real-world clinical practice. The methods used in studies establishing the efficacy of medications are at variance with the way disorders are treated in routine clinical practice. In particular, the rigorous inclusion and exclusion criteria used to select subjects for participation in efficacy studies potentially limits the generalizability of the results of these trials. Little is known about how much impact these inclusion and exclusion criteria have on the representativeness of subjects treated in efficacy trials. Data from the MIDAS project allow us to directly address this issue because we assessed patients presenting to a routine clinical practice with the same research methods used in treatment studies. This enabled us to apply exclusion criteria used in research studies of treatment efficacy to our sample of routine clinical practice patients.

In our first study of this issue we examined the representativeness of antidepressant efficacy trials by applying a hypothetical set of exclusion criteria to a large sample ($N = 346$) of depressed outpatients (Zimmerman et al. 2002b). We were limited to using a hypothetical set of exclusion criteria because of the lack of consensus in exclusion criteria used in efficacy studies. Approximately one-sixth of the 346 depressed patients would have been excluded from an efficacy trial because they had a bipolar or psychotic subtype of depression. In the remaining 293 outpatients with nonpsychotic, unipolar MDD the presence of a comorbid psychiatric disorder, insufficient severity of depressive symptoms, and current suicidal ideation would have excluded 86.4% of patients from an antidepressant efficacy trial.

In a subsequent study we reviewed the psychiatric exclusion criteria used in 39 recently published antidepressant efficacy trials and illustrated the impact different sets of exclusion criteria have on the generalizability of efficacy trials (M. Zimmerman et al., unpublished observations, 2003). We applied the exclusion criteria used in 35 of these studies to the depressed patients evaluated in the MIDAS project. This allowed us not only to examine the generalizability of each study but also to appreciate the range of generalizability between studies. Figure 2–3 illustrates the percentage of depressed patients seen in the MIDAS project who would have been excluded from each study. The percentage of patients who would have been excluded ranged from 0% to 95.0% (mean, 65.8%). In approximately half of the studies more than 70% of the depressed patients treated in our practice would not have qualified for the efficacy study. These findings indicate that there is wide variability in the exclusion criteria employed in antidepressant efficacy trials and that only a minority of depressed patients are likely to be eligible for most antidepressant efficacy trials.

Unanswered Questions

The results from the MIDAS project—along with the recently published studies of diagnosis in routine clinical practice from Pittsburgh, Texas, and Los Angeles—bring to the forefront the problem with diagnosis in routine clinical practice. It is perhaps not surprising that this problem has received greater attention in the past decade, because clinicians are struggling to conduct diagnostic evaluations more efficiently in the face of declining reimbursement rates. Conversations with many practicing psychiatrists in Rhode Island indicate that they complete their evaluations, including the write-up, in 30–45 minutes. This is consistent with the description of clinicians' practices in the report by Basco and colleagues (2000). The frequency of missed diagnoses, and possibly even misdiagnoses, should be expected to increase when insufficient time is allotted to the diagnostic examination.

Some important issues that should be addressed are what these findings suggest about the community standard of care in making psychiatric diagnoses, and whether and how the standard of care should be changed. Structured research diagnostic interviews are considered the diagnostic gold standard, albeit an imperfect one. In most contemporary research studies, diagnoses are based on these interview schedules. Judged against this standard, the Pittsburgh, Texas, Rhode Island, and

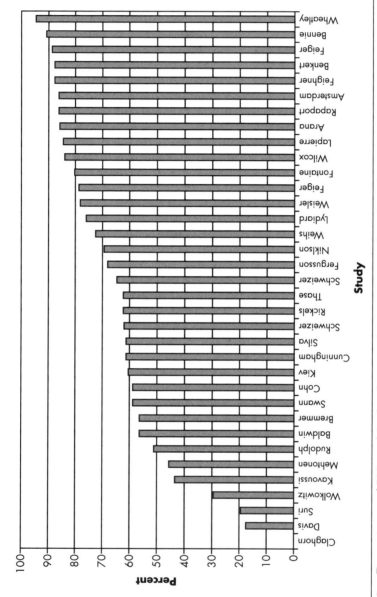

Figure 2–3. Percentages of 503 nonbipolar depressed patients treated in clinical practice in the Methods to Improve Diagnostic Assessment and Services (MIDAS) project who would have been excluded from 35 antidepressant efficacy trials based on the exclusion criteria for each trial.

Los Angeles studies suggest that clinicians are not doing a very good job.

Are these findings any cause for alarm? That is a difficult question to answer, because no research has yet examined the clinical significance of the gap between researchers' and clinicians' diagnostic practices. Specifically, we are not aware of any studies that have addressed the important question of whether the more accurate and comprehensive research diagnostic evaluations improve outcomes. In fact, one could argue that patients' outcomes are *not* more likely to be worse, even if diagnoses are missed, because of the broad spectrum of activity of the new generation of antidepressant medication. Clinicians currently have at their disposal pharmacological agents with broad-based efficacy; consequently, diagnostic error might not be important. Medications such as selective serotonin reuptake inhibitors have been found to be effective for depression, almost all anxiety disorders, eating disorders, impulse control disorders, substance use disorders, attention-deficit disorder, and some somatoform disorders. In short, most of the disorders for which individuals seek outpatient care have been found to be responsive to at least one of the new generation of antidepressant medications. Therefore, it is possible that accurate and comprehensive DSM-IV diagnoses are not critical after gross diagnostic class distinctions (e.g., psychotic disorder versus mood disorder) are made. This is consistent with the results of a survey of psychiatrists' attitudes about DSM-III and DSM-III-R conducted 10 years ago (Zimmerman et al. 1993). In that survey only a minority of psychiatrists rated DSM as being very important for treatment planning, determining prognosis, patient management, and understanding patients' problems.

Nevertheless, on common-sense grounds it seems logical that greater diagnostic accuracy will improve outcome. If the clinician is unaware of the presence of a comorbid condition, it seems unlikely that that condition will be successfully treated. More complete and accurate diagnostic evaluations might influence whether a medication is prescribed (e.g., an antidepressant is more likely to be prescribed if the patient is diagnosed with MDD instead of adjustment disorder), choice of medication (e.g., a selective serotonin reuptake inhibitor should be preferentially chosen for a depressed patient if a comorbid obsessive-compulsive disorder is recognized), the number of medications prescribed (e.g., a mood stabilizer should be added to an antidepressant in a depressed patient with a history of manic episodes), and the prescription of psychotherapy (e.g., cognitive-behavior therapy is preferred to supportive therapy for a patient diagnosed with a specific anxiety disorder instead of adjustment disorder).

One can also hypothesize that more complete and accurate knowledge of patients' psychiatric disorders might improve outcome independent of changes in treatment decisions. That is, better diagnostic practice may result in greater patient satisfaction with the diagnostic assessment, an improved alliance with the treating clinician, and consequently greater compliance with treatment and better outcome.

Whether or not improved diagnostic practice would result in improved outcome, it is important to recognize that diagnosis has more than one clinically relevant function. In addition to optimizing outcome, diagnosis is important for predicting treatment outcome. It would be expected that a greater percentage of the variance in outcome would be predicted by comprehensive evaluations than by clinical diagnoses. Again, this is an unstudied question.

If future research demonstrates that comprehensive research evaluations are better, either by improving outcome or by improving the prediction of outcome, then what can or should be done to change the standard of care regarding diagnostic evaluations? One possibility is the incorporation of semistructured diagnostic evaluations into routine clinical practice. One advantage to using instruments such as the SCID or the Mini-International Neuropsychiatric Interview (Sheehan et al. 1998) is that they ensure diagnostic thoroughness. Another is that they improve diagnostic reliability. Of course, it is unlikely that clinicians will adopt such measures without appropriate compensation for the additional time that will be needed to conduct the initial assessment. Even if greater reimbursement was forthcoming, it might prove difficult to change how clinicians conduct their initial diagnostic evaluation in the absence of compelling data warranting such a change. The data documenting the problems with current clinical diagnostic practice are clear and consistent; however, studies demonstrating the clinical effect size resulting from this problem have not yet been conducted. Consequently, it is premature to suggest that changes in the training of psychiatrists should be implemented in the absence of replicated research demonstrating the effect of less-than-optimal diagnostic performance on outcome.

In the meantime, until such studies are conducted, clinicians might want to consider whether one of the recently developed self-administered diagnostic screening questionnaires such as the PDSQ could be a useful adjunct to their unstructured diagnostic interview. Because clinicians often do not have the time to be as comprehensive as they would like, it was our hope that the measure could improve the efficiency of the diagnostic evaluation by guiding clinicians toward symptom areas that require more versus less assessment. The completion of paperwork before an initial evaluation is common in physicians' offices. The advantage of research measures over homegrown forms is that the psychometric and diagnostic properties of the research instruments have been established, thereby guiding the interpretation of the results. However, whether such measures as the PDSQ can improve diagnostic efficiency or accuracy, and consequently improve outcome, remains an empirical question.

In concluding, it is worth reflecting on the change in the discourse on diagnosis over the past 25 years. DSM-III, the first officially sanctioned diagnostic system to incorporate specified inclusion and exclusion criteria for psychiatric diagnosis, was published only 22 years ago. The empirical justification for the radical change in how psychiatric disorders were defined were the studies documenting problems with diagnostic reliability when diagnoses were based on earlier systems (Spitzer and Fleiss 1974) and other studies demonstrating that high levels of reliability could be achieved when diagnoses were derived from semistructured interviews and based on specific criteria (Spitzer et al. 1978). Validity was not so much an issue, except for some studies that demonstrated that the more narrow definition of schizophrenia proposed for DSM-III was more valid than the broader definition in DSM-II (Pope and Lipinski 1978). The clinical utility of the new diagnostic system was assumed, although improvement in patient outcomes was not the focus of attention.

Nearly a quarter of a century after the publication of DSM-III, recent research suggests that significant problems remain with psychiatric diagnosis in routine clinical practice. However, during the past two decades we have witnessed a revolution in the treatment of psychiatric disorders. Pharmacotherapies and psychotherapies have been repeatedly demonstrated to be effective for a wide range of disorders as defined in DSM-III, DSM-III-R, and DSM-IV. Consequently, it would seem more important now than 25 years ago that accurate diagnoses be made. It is to be hoped that the next generation of research on diagnosis (e.g., changes in diagnostic criteria or changes in diagnostic practice) will attend to the most salient aspect of psychiatric treatment: the outcome of care. Depending on the results of these studies, the integration of the assessment methods of researchers into routine clinical practice—which we have done in the MIDAS project—might become much more common later in this decade.

Thus far our work in the MIDAS project has focused on diagnostic precision and completeness, and our findings have raised the question of whether improvement in diagnostic practice will result in improved outcome or outcome prediction. Although a diagnostic determination is an important function of the intake evaluation, it is not its sole objective. Other integral functions of the intake evaluation include additional history taking (e.g., psychiatric history, prior treatment efforts, medical history, life events, social supports, coping style, family history, developmental history), education about the disorder and treatment options, establishment of a therapeutic alliance, and identification of obstacles of treatment. Striving for improved diagnostic practice should not come with a cost of sacrificing the important details of a patient's story so that a diagnosis (or diagnoses) can be made (Tucker 1998). It has been our experience during the past 6 years of the MIDAS project that the nondiagnostic functions of the initial evaluation are enhanced, rather than undermined, by good diagnostic practice. This too is an important question that can and should be the subject of empirical study.

References

American Psychiatric Association: Diagnostic and Statistical Manual of Mental Disorders, 2nd Edition. Washington, DC, American Psychiatric Association, 1968

American Psychiatric Association: Diagnostic and Statistical Manual of Mental Disorders, 3rd Edition. Washington, DC, American Psychiatric Association, 1980

American Psychiatric Association: Diagnostic and Statistical Manual of Mental Disorders, 3rd Edition, Revised. Washington, DC, American Psychiatric Association, 1987

American Psychiatric Association: Diagnostic and Statistical Manual of Mental Disorders, 4th Edition, Text Revision. Washington, DC, American Psychiatric Association, 2000

Basco MR, Bostic JQ, Davies D, et al: Methods to improve diagnostic accuracy in a community mental health setting. Am J Psychiatry 157:1599–1605, 2000

Beck AT, Rush AJ, Shaw BF, et al: Cognitive Therapy of Depression. New York, Guilford Press, 1979

Beck AT, Brown G, Epstein N, et al: An inventory for measuring clinical anxiety: psychometric properties. J Consult Clin Psychol 56:893–897, 1988

Berkson J: Limitations of the application of fourfold table analysis to hospital data. Biometric Bulletin 2:47–53, 1946

Butler RW, Mueser KT, Sprock J, et al: Positive symptoms of psychosis in posttraumatic stress disorder. Biol Psychiatry 39:839–844, 1996

Campbell DT, Fiske DW: Convergent and discriminant validation by the multitrait multi-method matrix. Psychol Bull 56:81–105, 1959

Coryell W, Zimmerman M: Progress in the classification of functional psychoses. Am J Psychiatry 144:1471–1474, 1987

Deering CG, Glover SG, Ready D, et al: Unique patterns of comorbidity in posttraumatic stress disorder from different sources of trauma. Compr Psychiatry 37:336–346, 1996

Endicott J, Spitzer RL: A diagnostic interview: the Schedule for Affective Disorders and Schizophrenia. Arch Gen Psychiatry 35:837–844, 1978

Endicott J, Andreasen N, Spitzer RL: Family History-Research Diagnostic Criteria (FH-RDC). Washington, DC, National Institute on Mental Health, 1978

Feighner JP, Robins E, Guze SB, et al: Diagnostic criteria for use in psychiatric research. Arch Gen Psychiatry 26:57–67, 1972

First M, Spitzer R, Gibbon M, Williams JB: Structured Clinical Interview for DSM-IV Axis I Disorders (SCID). New York, New York State Psychiatric Institute, 1995

Foa EB, Riggs DS, Dancu CV, et al: Reliability and validity of a brief instrument for assessing post-traumatic stress disorder. J Trauma Stress 6:459–473, 1993

Franklin CL, Zimmerman M: Posttraumatic stress disorder and major depressive disorder: investigating the role of overlapping symptoms in diagnostic comorbidity. J Nerv Ment Dis 189:548–551, 2001

Franklin CL, Sheeran T, Zimmerman M: Assessing trauma and trauma related syndromes in psychiatric outpatients. Psychological Assessment (in press)

Garner DM, Olmstead MP, Polivy J: Development and validation of a multidimensional eating disorder inventory for anorexia nervosa and bulimia. Int J Eat Disord 2:15–34, 1983

Green BL, Lindy JD, Grace MC, et al: Multiple diagnoses in posttraumatic stress disorder: the role of war stressors. J Nerv Ment Dis 177:329–335, 1989

Grunhaus L: Clinical and psychobiological characteristics of simultaneous panic disorder and major depression. Am J Psychiatry 145:1214–1221, 1988

Hamilton M: A rating scale for depression. J Neurol Neurosurg Psychiatry 23:56–62, 1960

Hodgson RJ, Rachman S: Obsessional compulsive complaints. Behav Res Ther 10:111–117, 1977

Hsiao JK, Bartko JJ, Potter WZ: Diagnosing diagnoses: receiver operating characteristic methods and psychiatry. Arch Gen Psychiatry 46:664–667, 1989

Hyler SE, Rieder RD, Williams JBW, et al: The Personality Diagnostic Questionnaire: development and preliminary results. J Personal Disord 2:229–237, 1988

Keller MB, Klerman GL, Lavori PW, et al: Long-term outcomes of episodes of major depression. JAMA 252:788–792, 1984

Kellner R: The Symptom Rating Test, in Assessment of Depression. Edited by Sartorius N, Ban TA. New York, Springer-Verlag, 1985

Kessler RC, McGonagle KA, Zhao S, et al: Lifetime and 12-month prevalence of DSM-III-R psychiatric disorders in the United States. Arch Gen Psychiatry 51:8–19, 1994

Kessler RC, Sonnega A, Bromet E, et al: Posttraumatic stress disorder in the National Comorbidity Survey. Arch Gen Psychiatry 52:1048–1060, 1995

Klerman GL, Vailant GE, Spitzer RL, et al: A debate on DSM-III. Am J Psychiatry 141:539–542, 1984

Koenigsberg HW, Kaplan RD, Gilmore MM, et al: The relationship between syndrome and personality disorder in DSM-III: experience with 2,462 patients. Am J Psychiatry 142:207–212, 1985

Kuhner C, Veiel HO: Psychometrische und diagnostiche Eigenschaften einer duetschsprachigen Version des Inventory to Diagnose Depression (IDD). Diagnostica 39:229–321, 1993

Leary MR: A brief version of the Fear of Negative Evaluation Scale. Pers Soc Psychol Bull 9:371–375, 1983

Loranger AW: The impact of DSM-III on diagnostic practice in a university hospital. Arch Gen Psychiatry 47:672–675, 1990

Marks IM, Mathews AM: Brief standard self-rating for phobic patients. Behav Res Ther 17:263–267, 1979

Maser JD, Cloninger CR: Comorbidity of Mood and Anxiety Disorders. Washington, DC, American Psychiatric Association, 1990

Melartin TK, Rytsala HJ, Leskela US, et al: Current comorbidity of psychiatric disorders among DSM-IV major depressive disorder patients in psychiatric care in the Vantaa Depression Study. J Clin Psychiatry 63:126–134, 2002

Meyer TJ, Miller ML, Metzger RL, et al: Development and validation of the Penn State Worry Questionnaire. Behav Res Ther 28:487–495, 1990

Mezzich JE, Fabrega H, Coffman GA, et al: DSM-III disorders in a large sample of psychiatric patients: frequency and specificity of diagnoses. Am J Psychiatry 146:212–219, 1989

Miller PR, Dasher R, Collins R, et al: Inpatient diagnostic assessments: 1. Accuracy of structured vs. unstructured interviews. Psychiatry Res 105:255–264, 2001

Millon T: Manual for the Millon Clinical Multiaxial Inventory-III (MCMI-III). Minneapolis, MN, National Computer Systems, 1994

Mossman D, Somoza E: Maximizing diagnostic information from the dexamethasone suppression test. Arch Gen Psychiatry 46:653–660, 1989

Noyes R, Reich J, Christiansen J, et al: Outcome of panic disorder. Arch Gen Psychiatry 47:809–818, 1990

Oldham JM, Skodol AE: Personality disorders in the public sector. Hosp Community Psychiatry 42:481–487, 1991

Olfson M, Marcus SC, Druss B, et al: National trends in the outpatient treatment of depression. JAMA 287:203–209, 2002

Othmer E, DeSouza C: A screening test for somatization disorder (hysteria). Am J Psychiatry 1142:1146–1149, 1985

Pfohl B, Stangl D, Zimmerman M: The implications of DSM-III personality disorders for patients with major depression. J Affect Disord 7:309–318, 1984

Pfohl B, Blum N, Zimmerman M: Structured Interview for DSM-IV Personality. Washington, DC, American Psychiatric Press, 1997

Phillips KA: Body dysmorphic disorder: the distress of imagined ugliness. Am J Psychiatry 148:1138–1149, 1991

Phillips KA, McElroy SL, Keck PE, et al: Body dysmorphic disorder: 30 cases of imagined ugliness. Am J Psychiatry 150:302–308, 1993

Phillips KA, McElroy SL, Keck PE, et al: A comparison of delusional and nondelusional body dysmorphic disorder in 100 cases. Psychopharmacol Bull 30:179–186, 1994

Pilowsky I: Dimensions of hypochondriasis. Br J Psychiatry 113:89–93, 1967

Pope HG, Lipinski JF: Diagnosis in schizophrenia and manic-depressive illness. Arch Gen Psychiatry 35:811–828, 1978

Posternak MA, Zimmerman M: Switching versus augmentation: a prospective, naturalistic comparison in depressed, treatment-resistant patients. J Clin Psychiatry 62:135–142, 2001

Posternak MA, Zimmerman M, Solomon DA: Integrating outcomes research into clinical practice: a pilot study. Psychiatr Serv 53:335–336, 2002

Pribor EF, Dinwiddie SH: Psychiatric correlates of incest in childhood. Am J Psychiatry 149:52–56, 1992

Robins LN, Locke BZ, Regier DA: An overview of psychiatric disorders in America, in Psychiatric Disorders in America: The Epidemiologic Catchment Study. Edited by Robins LN, Regier DA. New York, Free Press, 1991, pp 328–366

Roszell DK, McFall ME, Malas KL: Frequency of symptoms and concurrent psychiatric disorder in Vietnam veterans with chronic PTSD. Hosp Community Psychiatry 42:293–296, 1991

Sabshin M: Comorbidity: a central concern of psychiatry in the 1990s. Hosp Community Psychiatry 42:345, 1991

Sanderson WC, Moran ME, Kocsis JH, et al: Syndrome comorbidity in patients with major depression or dysthymia: prevalence and temporal relationships. Am J Psychiatry 147:1025–1028, 1990

Selzer ML: The Michigan Alcoholism Screening Test: the quest for a new diagnostic instrument. Am J Psychiatry 127:1653–1658, 1971

Shear MK, Greeno C, Kang J, et al: Diagnosis of nonpsychotic patients in community clinics. Am J Psychiatry 157:581–587, 2000

Sheehan DV, LeCrubier Y, Sheehan KH, et al: The Mini-International Neuropsychiatric Interview (M.I.N.I.): The development and validation of a structured diagnostic psychiatric interview for DSM-IV and ICD-10. J Clin Psychiatry 59 (suppl. 20):22–33, 1998

Shugar G, Schertzer S, Toner BB, et al: Development, use, and factor analysis of a self-report inventory for mania. Compr Psychiatry 33:325–331, 1992

Sierles FS, Chen JJ, McFarland RE, et al: Posttraumatic stress disorder and concurrent psychiatric illness: a preliminary report. Am J Psychiatry 140:1177–1179, 1983

Skinner HA: The Drug Abuse Screening Test. Addict Behav 7:363–371, 1982

Spitzer R, Fleiss J: A re-analysis of the reliability of psychiatric diagnosis. Br J Psychiatry 125:341–347, 1974

Spitzer RL, Endicott J, Robins E: Research diagnostic criteria: rationale and reliability. Arch Gen Psychiatry 35:773–782, 1978

Stangl D, Pfohl G, Zimmerman M, et al: A structured interview for the DSM-III personality disorders. Arch Gen Psychiatry 42:591–596, 1985

Stangler RS, Printz AM: DSM-III: Psychiatric diagnosis in a university population. Am J Psychiatry 137:937–940, 1979

Swartz M, Hughes D, George L, et al: Developing a screening index for community studies of somatization disorder. J Psychiatr Res 20:335–343, 1986

Thelen MH, Farmer J, Wonderlich S, et al: A revision of the Bulimia Test: the BULIT-R. Psychol Assess 3:119–124, 1991

Thelen MH, Mintz LB, Vander Wal JS: The bulimia test-revised: validation with DSM-IV criteria for bulimia nervosa. Psychol Assess 8:219–221, 1996

Tucker GJ: Putting DSM-IV in perspective. Am J Psychiatry 155:159–161, 1998

Zimmerman M, Chelminski I: Generalized anxiety disorder in patients with major depressive disorder: is DSM-IV's hierarchy correct? American Journal of Psychiatry (in press)

Zimmerman M, Coryell W: The validity of a self-report questionnaire for diagnosing major depressive disorder. Arch Gen Psychiatry 45:738–740, 1988

Zimmerman M, Coryell WH: DSM-III personality disorder dimensions. J Nerv Ment Dis 178:686–692, 1990

Zimmerman M, Coryell W: Screening for major depressive disorder in the community: a comparison of measures. Psychol Assess 6:71–74, 1994

Zimmerman M, Mattia JI: Body dysmorphic disorder in psychiatric outpatients: recognition, prevalence, comorbidity, demographic, and clinical correlates. Compr Psychiatry 39:265–270, 1998

Zimmerman M, Mattia JI: Axis I diagnostic comorbidity and borderline personality disorder. Compr Psychiatry 40:245–252, 1999a

Zimmerman M, Mattia JI: Differences between clinical and research practice in diagnosing borderline personality disorder. Am J Psychiatry 156:1570–1574, 1999b

Zimmerman M, Mattia JI: Is posttraumatic stress disorder underdiagnosed in routine clinical settings? J Nerv Ment Dis 187:420–428, 1999c

Zimmerman M, Mattia JI: Psychiatric diagnosis in clinical practice: is comorbidity being missed? Compr Psychiatry 40:182–191, 1999d

Zimmerman M, Mattia JI: Psychotic subtyping of major depressive disorder and posttraumatic stress disorder. J Clin Psychiatry 60:311–314, 1999e

Zimmerman M, Mattia JI: The reliability and validity of a screening questionnaire for 13 DSM-IV Axis I disorders (the Psychiatric Diagnostic Screening Questionnaire) in psychiatric outpatients. J Clin Psychiatry 60:677–683, 1999f

Zimmerman M, Mattia JI: Principal and additional DSM-IV disorders for which outpatients seek treatment. Psychiatr Serv 51:1299–1304, 2000

Zimmerman M, Mattia JI: The Psychiatric Diagnostic Screening Questionnaire: development, reliability and validity. Compr Psychiatry 42:175–189, 2001a

Zimmerman M, Mattia JI: A self-report scale to help make psychiatric diagnoses: the Psychiatric Diagnostic Screening Questionnaire (PDSQ). Arch Gen Psychiatry 58:787–794, 2001b

Zimmerman M, Coryell W, Corenthal C, et al: A self-report scale to diagnose major depression disorder. Arch Gen Psychiatry 43:1076–1081, 1986a

Zimmerman M, Coryell W, Pfohl B, et al: The validity of four definitions of endogenous depression. Arch Gen Psychiatry 43:234–244, 1986b

Zimmerman M, Pfohl B, Coryell WH, et al: Major depression and personality disorder. J Affect Disord 22:199–210, 1991

Zimmerman M, Jampala VC, Sierles FS, et al: DSM-III and DSM-III-R: what are American psychiatrists using and why? Compr Psychiatry 34:365–374, 1993

Zimmerman M, Chelminski I, McDermut W: Major depressive disorder and Axis I diagnostic comorbidity. J Clin Psychiatry 63:187–193, 2002a

Zimmerman M, Mattia JI, Posternak MA: Are subjects in pharmacological treatment trials of depression representative of patients in routine clinical practice? Am J Psychiatry 159:469–473, 2002b

Chapter 3

Use of Structured Diagnostic Interviews in Clinical Child Psychiatric Practice

Christopher P. Lucas, M.D., M.P.H.

To make a psychiatric diagnosis in a child, a clinician must 1) know the phenomenology of the condition; 2) carry out a systematic inquiry with the patient or with a knowledgeable second informant about the child's past and current behavior, emotions, and thoughts; 3) directly observe the patient's behavior and language; and, where appropriate, 4) interpret the results of specific tests of language, academic ability, or intelligence. Until recently, each of these elements has required professional expertise.

The development of operationalized, criterion-based diagnostic systems has promoted the creation of structured diagnostic interviews, which allow lay interviewers with no clinical training to elicit sufficient defining information for many symptoms and diagnoses. Although skilled inquiry about complex and poorly understood phenomenology, expert observation of behavior, interpretation of language cues, and the administration of specialized tests remain the province of the clinician, not all diagnoses require such expertise. Clinical observation and clinically astute and adaptive questioning may be crucial in the differential diagnosis of schizophrenia, for example, but may be less important for the diagnosis of common disorders characterized by overt behaviors that are rarely witnessed by a clinician.

Knowledge about symptoms cannot provide all the information necessary for effective treatment planning or for the understanding of causation; however, the comprehensive and systematic assessment of symptoms is an essential part of any clinical evaluation of children and adolescents. Although they are used extensively in research protocols, standardized diagnostic assessments are rarely part of the evaluation process in most clinical outpatient services. This has principally been due to the fact that many assessment procedures require clinical expertise that is arguably better spent on the routine complex clinical assessment that incorporates information about symptoms, context, and reactive or personality style that is essential for treatment planning.

Problems With Clinical Interviewing

Despite its strengths, the unstructured clinical interview has many flaws and fallibilities (see Kendell 1975) that can be addressed by a structured diagnostic interview. These include the following:

- **Variable structure.** Clinicians differ in the way they structure diagnostic interviews with patients. Clinicians often make up their minds about the potential diagnosis of a patient within the first 5 minutes of an interview, based on very limited information (chiefly the presenting complaint) and then proceed to ask a series of questions that tend to confirm the presence of that diagnostic entity, often to the extent of ignoring conflicting evidence (Elstein et al. 1972; Kendell 1973; Simon et al. 1971). Other clinicians may be constantly deflected by the receipt of new information, altering their line of questioning and area of symptomatic and functional inquiry, with the result that they never fully explore any specific diagnostic area (Gauron and Dickinson 1966a).
- **Variable coverage of symptoms and problems.** The nature of a clinical interview has been shown to preclude an exhaustive examination of all possible symptoms. Rare or socially embarrassing items are frequently overlooked (Bagley and Genius 1991; Beck et al. 1988; Greist et al. 1973; Levine et al. 1989; R.W. Lucas et al. 1977). Clinicians often have very little idea of the true probabilities of symptom-disease relationships

(Gauron and Dickinson 1966a; Leaper et al. 1972), and this can produce erratic exploration or abandonment of inquiry into potentially important diagnostic domains.

- **Variable effect of personal characteristics and the assessment environment.** The nonclinical characteristics of a patient—such as race, gender, and age—can affect how clinicians conduct a clinical interview, leading them to focus on certain issues or, more importantly, to avoid others (Burgoyne 1977; Gauron and Dickinson 1966b). For example, if it is believed that males do not experience eating disorders, then exploration of weight, eating, and attitudes to body shape may be cursory. Similarly, preconceptions about age and depression may lead to underidentification of major depressive disorder in prepubertal children. It has also been shown that certain settings (e.g., juvenile justice locations) can influence the nature and range of diagnoses that are inquired about (Kendell 1975), which can result in a decreased likelihood that anxiety and mood disorders will be recognized in delinquent adolescents.

- **Inconsistent application of diagnostic criteria.** The advent of frequently changing criterion-based diagnostic systems—such as DSM-III (American Psychiatric Association 1980), DSM-III-R (American Psychiatric Association 1987), DSM-IV (American Psychiatric Association 1994), DSM-IV-TR (American Psychiatric Association 2000), and the International Classification of Diseases, 10th Edition (ICD-10) (World Health Organization 1993)—may have introduced a new source of clinical unreliability. It is almost impossible for clinicians to remember numerous complex and lengthy lists of diagnostic criteria, and many child psychiatrists do not routinely consult or check diagnostic manuals (Setterberg et al. 1991). It is no insult to clinicians to question the ability of even the most able and diligent among them to accurately apply diagnostic criteria and decision trees, organize and retain diagnostic logic, eliminate bias, and use diagnostic labels in the way they were intended to be used.

Many of these problems can be obviated by the use of the same standardized interviewing techniques that have gained wide acceptance in clinical and epidemiological research.

Semistructured Diagnostic Interviews

The first historical response by the research community to the problems of unreliable clinical diagnostic assessments was to devise semistructured interviews that guided clinicians with required questions and glossary definitions for constructs such as *panic attack* or *anhedonia*. These interviews, derived from the Present State Examination (Wing et al. 1974) and the Isle of Wight interview (Graham and Rutter 1968), are less structured and use clinicians or extensively trained paraprofessional people as interviewers. This is because these semistructured assessments require the interviewers to make judgments as to whether a subject meets a glossary-defined symptom pattern, criterion threshold, or point on a simple continuous scale. Examples of such instruments in child and adolescent psychiatry are the Child and Adolescent Psychiatric Assessment (CAPA) (Angold et al. 1995) or the various incarnations of the Schedule for Affective Disorders and Schizophrenia for School-Aged Children (K-SADS) (Puig-Antich and Chambers 1978).

In semistructured interviewing, the interviewer has the freedom to change the order or wording of questions and will often determine whether a subject has a particular symptom or construct (e.g., depressed mood) by the degree to which the subject's responses match an internally held or externally defined glossary definition. Additional time and expense may result from the need to record the interview and to have post-hoc editing by an interview supervisor to ensure interrater reliability.

Fully Structured Diagnostic Interviews

In epidemiological research there is a particular need for reliable measures that can be given to a large number of subjects at lower cost than can be achieved with methods that require clinicians or phenomenal amounts of training, supervision, and postinterview coding and editing. These cost-efficiency requirements—which mirror the needs of understaffed clinical providers of services for children and adolescents—led to the development of structured diagnostic interviews such as the Diagnostic Interview Schedule for Children (DISC) developed by the National Institute of Mental Health (see Shaffer et al. 1996) and the Diagnostic Interview for Children and Adolescents (Herjanic and Reich 1982)

A structured diagnostic interview is best viewed as a precise script that obtains clinically relevant information through carefully worded and ordered questions that are administered to the informant as written. Typically, answers given to these questions are restricted to a few predefined alternatives (usually "yes" or "no"). The only role of the interviewer is to accurately and faithfully read the question, determine the subject's comprehension, and record the answer that is given.

The authors of these structured measures attempted to embody all the required elements that a clinician would use in judging a symptom, criterion, or diagnosis to be present or absent by a complex series of contingent questions, the answers to which are taken at face value (Anthony et al. 1985). Although the predefined questions and limited response options of structured diagnostic interviews resemble those of symptom questionnaires such as the Child Behavior Checklist (Achenbach and Edelbrock 1983) or the Achenbach-Conners-Quay Behavior Checklist (Achenbach et al. 1993), questionnaires usually obtain less-detailed information about symptoms and have a simpler, more linear format—that is, one question is followed by the next with few if any branches or skips. In contrast, the typical structured diagnostic interview includes many contingencies that are used to determine whether a reported symptom is *clinically* significant by matching the criteria laid down in the diagnostic classification systems.

Although the contingencies resemble the normal iterative process of the clinical interview, they are too complex for the interviewee to navigate without assistance. As a result, the order and content of the questions need to be directed by a trained interviewer or by a computer. With advances in computer technology, the operational differences between questionnaires and structured diagnostic interviews have narrowed. Highly complex diagnostic interviews can now be directed by a computer instead of an interviewer and, like questionnaires, can be self-completed. Similarly, standardized responses can be readily extracted to provide scales for use in dimensional analyses, traditionally the province of questionnaires.

Relative Advantages of Semistructured and Structured Diagnostic Interviews

The main advantages of the structured approach of the DISC over the semistructured methodology of the K-SADS or the CAPA are that the DISC has much greater potential for standardization and reliability and is inherently less expensive to use. The interview content (question wording, logical flow, and scoring algorithms) is transparent and fixed. With repeated testing and modification it is hoped one can hope that new versions of the interview better approximate constructs defined by diagnostic criteria. By contrast, the reliability and validity of a semistructured interview is subject to variations in skill, thoroughness, quality of training, and supervision (Angold and Costello 1995). The rigid script of the DISC and the limited range of response options make it much easier to computerize, with consequent efficiencies in data management.

There are several potential disadvantages of the fully structured approach. The structured approach typified by the DISC brings with it a reduced ability to determine whether the subject understands the question or has a shared definition of the construct being probed. In contrast, a clinician using the K-SADS, for example, can repeat and rephrase a question to optimize comprehension, ask the subject for examples, and use clinical experience to check that the example given matches the target symptom. Semistructured interviews offer a better opportunity to elicit atypical phenomena because they permit different methods of eliciting and synthesizing information about symptoms that may be hard to define succinctly. For a complex symptom to be accurately elicited and classified may require that the subject be asked to describe the symptom at greater length—something that is generally not possible with the DISC. Time savings (although with the risks discussed above) are possible because the interviewer can use his or her clinical judgment to cut short a line of questioning and skip to a more fruitful area in the interview.

The Diagnostic Interview Schedule for Children

The first version of the Diagnostic Interview Schedule for Children, the DISC-1 (Costello et al. 1984), was based on DSM-III. Its design included many open-ended questions that required post-interview coding. The instrument was designed to be highly sensitive, with generally low thresholds for defining a behavior or a feeling as abnormal. A validity study (Costello et al. 1984) showed what appeared to be implausibly high prevalence rates and poor correspondence between DISC diagnoses and case conference diagnoses, although this finding was probably more a reflection of the poor agreement between informants.

The next version of the instrument, the DISC-R (largely DSM-III-R compatible), was developed by modifying questions found to be unreliable in the Costello sample and questions that had a very high prevalence rate in a nonreferred community population (Shaffer et al. 1993). As with the DISC-R, field trial data were used to modify and test the next version of the interview, the DISC-2.1, and subsequently the DISC-2.3 (Shaffer et al. 1996). The DISC-2.1 was field tested in a four-site study, the Methods for Epidemiology of Child and Adolescent Mental Disorders (MECA) study (see Lahey et al. 1996). The DISC-2.3, which appeared in 1991, was prepared with consultation from the diagnostic committee of the MECA study based on data and interviewer feedback from the DISC-2.1 field trial and sensitivity studies. The DISC-2.3 was the first DISC that was computerized for ease of administration.

Further field trials were used to estimate the test-retest reliability of DISC-2.3 diagnoses. In each revision of the original DISC (Edelbrock et al. 1985)—DISC-R (Schwab-Stone et al. 1993), DISC 2.1 (Jensen et al. 1995; Roberts et al. 1996), and DISC 2.3 (Schwab-Stone et al. 1996)—diagnostic reliability improved modestly (Table 3–1).

When comparing psychometric studies, however, it is important to bear in mind that the results from community studies will always show lower reliability than those derived from clinical populations and that studies that exclude the youngest children

Table 3–1. Test-retest reliability of early versions of the Diagnostic Interview Schedule for Children (DISC)

	DISC[a]		DISC-R[b]		DISC 2.1[c]		DISC 2.1[d]	DISC 2.1[c]		DISC 2.3[e]	
	Parent ICC	Child ICC	Parent κ	Child κ	Parent κ	Child κ	Child κ	Parent κ	Child κ	Parent κ	Child κ
Anxiety	0.78	0.62	—	0.72	0.58	0.39	0.57	0.40	0.30	0.45	0.27
MDD	0.80	0.64	0.72	0.77	0.69	0.38	0.50	0.00	0.29	0.55	0.37
ADHD	0.84	0.67	0.55	—	0.69	0.59	0.47	0.57	0.43	0.60	0.10
ODD	0.80	0.73	0.87	0.16	0.67	0.46	0.67	0.65	0.23	0.68	0.18
CD	0.86	0.73	0.87	0.55	0.70	0.86	0.56	0.66	0.60	0.56	0.64
Setting	Clinical		Clinical		Clinical		Clinical	Community		Community	
Age	6–18 years		11–17 years		9–17 years		12–17 years	9–17 years		9–17 years	

Note. ICC=intraclass correlation coefficient; MDD=major depressive disorder; ADHD=attention-deficit/hyperactivity disorder; ODD=oppositional defiant disorder; CD=conduct disorder.
[a]Data from Edelbrock et al. 1985.
[b]Data from Schwab-Stone et al. 1993.
[c]Data from Jensen et al. 1995.
[d]Data from Roberts et al. 1996.
[e]Data from Schwab-Stone et al. 1996.

from their sample will also tend to achieve better reliability. In addition, results expressed as intraclass correlation coefficients (Shrout and Fleiss 1979) with symptom or criterion scale scores will produce higher values (on the order of +0.2) than diagnostic κ values (Cohen 1960) calculated from the same data.

The most recent study of the criterion validity of the NIMH DISC (Schwab-Stone et al. 1996) was carried out as part of the MECA study (Lahey et al. 1996) and used the DSM-III-R version of the interview (DISC-2.3). Using a design that permitted several comparisons of DISC-generated diagnoses based on clinician symptom rating scales, 247 youths, ages 9–18 years, were selected from the 1,285 parent-youth pairs that constituted the four-site MECA sample. Subjects who screened positive for any of the five diagnostic areas under investigation in the validity study (attention-deficit/hyperactivity disorder, oppositional defiant disorder, conduct disorder, depressive disorder, and the major anxiety disorders) were recruited, as were a comparable number of subjects who screened negative. After receiving a conventional lay-administered DISC, each youth and primary caregiver were separately reinterviewed by a clinician using the DISC. This was followed by a clinical-style interview in which the clinician rated the presence of symptoms and impairment and reexamined a number of symptoms and diagnoses that had secretly been flagged by the clinician during the course of the DISC interview as being worthy of further inquiry. Computer algorithms then combined this information into diagnoses using comparable rules for both DISC and clinical-rating diagnoses.

In general, the DISC showed moderate to good validity across a number of diagnoses (Table 3–2). Apart from a few notable exceptions (major depressive disorder and separation anxiety disorder), the validity of youth-derived DISC diagnoses was worse than that of the parent report. The agreement between a clinician-administered DISC (using standard DISC interviewing practices) and clinician ratings, for both youth and parent versions, was generally much better than agreement between two DISC interviews on the same subject separated by an interval. The test-retest paradigm showed significant evidence of attenuation of symptom reports (Jensen et al. 1995). Having clinicians

Table 3–2. Validity of clinician-administered DISC-2.3 diagnoses versus diagnoses from clinician symptom ratings

	Parent κ	Youth κ
ADHD	0.72	0.27
ODD	0.59	0.54
CD	0.74	0.77
MDD	0.60	0.79
Dysthymia	0.35	0.54
Overanxious disorder	0.62	0.23
Separation anxiety	0.29	0.59
Social phobia	0.53	0.45

Note. DISC=Diagnostic Interview Schedule for Children; ADHD=attention-deficit/hyperactivity disorder; ODD=oppositional defiant disorder; CD=conduct disorder; MDD=major depressive disorder.
Source. Adapted from Schwab-Stone et al. 1996.

rate dubious reports during the course of the DISC interview somewhat mitigated the effects of the passage of time on the validation assessment, but test-retest reliability must place a ceiling on observed DISC-clinician concordance because agreement with the reference procedure cannot be higher than with the same measure given on two separate occasions. This design is superior to having clinicians perform another semistructured interview after administering the DISC, because the reference procedure frequently has poor reliability (Piacentini et al. 1993) and introduces a systematic order effect (C.P. Lucas 1992).

DSM-IV Versions of the DISC

Generic (Epidemiological) DISC-IV

A major revision of the DISC (the Generic DISC-IV) (Shaffer et al. 2000) was completed in April 1997. It differed from the DISC-2.3 by including an assessment of DSM-IV and ICD-10 criteria, substituting a double time frame (1 month and 1 year) for the single 6-month time frame, including an optional module for lifetime diagnosis, and having more precise probing for episode onset. Based on experience from the MECA study and a series of item-specific analyses (Fallon and Schwab-Stone 1994; C.P. Lucas et al. 1999), further revisions to the DISC-IV included 1) identifying and revising particularly unreliable questions, 2) avoiding contingent questions with vague wording, 3) increasing use of categorical responses rather than asking for open-ended responses, 4) avoiding questions with multiple constructs, 5) limiting question length to fewer than 20 words whenever possible, and 6) writing items that sound more pathological to reduce "yea saying."

Reliability of the DISC-IV. A complete report on the test-retest reliability of the English version of the DISC-IV in clinical and community samples is in preparation (William Narrow, personal communication, February 2002); partial results based on one of the clinical samples (the Tri-site Study) were included in a report by Shaffer et al. (2000).

The sample for the Tri-site Study was 88 children ages 9–17 years (mean age, 12.6 years) recruited from one of four child psychiatry outpatient clinics; 57% of the children were male and 60% were nonwhite (including Hispanic). Interviewers were blind to clinical diagnosis and to results of all other DISC interviews (four interviewers were used for each parent-child pair). The interval between the first and second administrations of the DISC was 3–10 days; the mean interval was 6.6 days. DISC interviewers were trained for 2–4 days on DISC administration, and families were paid for their participation.

The κ statistic was used to evaluate the reliability of diagnoses when the number of cases was sufficient. Test-retest reliability for diagnoses is presented in Table 3–3, as is test-retest reliability for symptom and criterion scales. The reliability of scales was calculated using intraclass correlation coefficients. Overall, the Generic DISC-IV showed acceptable reliability for most diagnoses, with κ values ranging from fair to excellent. In general, the parent interview (DISC-P) was more reliable than the youth interview (DISC-Y); exceptions to this were conduct disorder (κ=0.69 for the DISC-Y versus κ=0.45 for the DISC-P) and major depression (κ=0.78 for the DISC-Y versus κ=0.69 for the DISC-P), for which the DISC-Y was more reliable. The DISC-Y

Table 3–3. Test-retest reliability of the Generic DISC-IV in a clinical sample

	Youth informant (DISC-Y)				Parent informant (DISC-P)			
	Diagnosis		Scales		Diagnosis		Scales	
			Criteria	Symptoms			Criteria	Symptoms
			ICC				ICC	
	n	κ			n	κ		
ADD	81	0.42	0.70	0.60	82	0.77	0.90	0.83
ODD	80	0.51	0.27	0.56	82	0.52	0.29	0.81
CD	79	0.69	0.73	0.79	82	0.45	0.71	0.87
Specific phobia	81	0.41	0.55	0.66	84	0.54	0.83	0.82
Social phobia	82	0.25	0.71	0.70	83	0.54	0.70	0.78
Separation anxiety	82	0.42	0.63	0.53	83	0.58	0.79	0.80
Generalized anxiety disorder	82	—	0.29	0.56	83	0.65	0.72	0.72
Major depression	82	0.78	0.81	0.61	83	0.69	0.82	0.82

Note. DISC=Diagnostic Interview Schedule for Children; ADD=attention-deficit disorder; ODD=oppositional defiant disorder; CD=conduct disorder.

Source. Adapted from Shaffer et al. 2000.

had poor reliability for social phobia ($\kappa=0.25$). The reliability of the symptom and criterion scales was better (often substantially) than that for most diagnoses, regardless of informant. Symptom scale reliability (intraclass correlation coefficient) ranged from 0.53 to 0.87 and, for all but one of the DISC-P symptom scales, was excellent.

Present State DISC

The Present State version of the DISC-IV has recently been developed (C.P. Lucas et al. 1997) and is thought to be of greater utility and appeal to clinicians. It differs from the Generic DISC-IV in asking mainly about the past 4 weeks (unless the minimum duration for disorder diagnosis required by DSM-IV is greater than 4 weeks), uses questions primarily in the present tense, and has simpler methods of assessing co-occurrence of symptoms.

Computerized Diagnostic Interview Schedule for Children

Recent versions of the DISC (the Generic DISC-IV and Present State DISC) have been computerized for interviewer administration. In the computerized versions, the computer handles the often complex rules controlling question wording, question flow, and scoring. With this development, the Computerized Diagnostic Interview Schedule for Children (C-DISC) has become the most widely used and studied child psychiatric interview.

Despite the research origins of the C-DISC, the benefits of a computer program that does not require a clinician and that provides comprehensive diagnostic coverage have made this research tool increasingly attractive to providers of clinical services. Unlike human interviewers—who frequently omit questions in error, read out the wrong question, or misread questions (Bradburn and Sudman 1979)—the computer is able to precisely follow a complex branching structure of questioning, avoiding redundant or inappropriate questioning, and can then produce an instant, accurate printed diagnostic report.

However, despite computerization, the continued need for trained interviewers to read out the questions and enter the interview responses has hindered the widespread adoption of the

C-DISC to provide low-cost routine standardized diagnostic assessment in psychiatric clinics and other settings where mental health services are provided.

Voice DISC

Advances in technology (Berg et al. 1992) have now made it possible to have questions read aloud by a computer (using a natural human voice) while the text is displayed on screen. This has enabled the creation of computer-assisted self-interview with audio (audio-CASI) versions of the C-DISC, the first of which is the Voice DISC. This software makes it practical for subjects, who may have limited reading skills, to complete a complex diagnostic interview independently. Of particular benefit in the search for standardization and increased reliability is that the computer will always read out each question in exactly the same way, with optimal and identical tonal emphasis. Privacy can be enhanced by delivering the spoken questions through headphones.

There are a number of potential advantages for use of the Voice DISC in child and adolescent clinical settings. Automated assessments are cost-effective (Erdman et al. 1985) and rapid, require little training of those who will administer them, and have high acceptability (Berg et al. 1992; Coddington and King 1972; Sawyer et al. 1991). In contrast to a clinical interviewer, the computer program will always ask the same questions in the same order (given the same responses) and will apply diagnostic criteria (algorithms) in a predictable and consistent fashion.

The traditional clinician's assessment synthesizes information from a variety of sources, most commonly the parent and the child. This can be emulated by the scoring algorithms for the DISC, which combines symptomatic information from parent and child to arrive at a diagnosis. It has been shown that diagnoses derived in this way, using a combined algorithm, have greater reliability and validity than those derived from any one informant alone (Jensen et al. 1995).

Many clinicians use specific symptom scales to measure severity and to monitor change as the result of treatment. The criterion-based specific symptom scales that can be derived from the DISC have an advantage over the most commonly used empirically derived rating scales, such as the Youth Self Report (Achenbach and Edelbrock 1987), because they reflect symptoms that have been found to be more clinically salient and constructs that have greater treatment specificity.

Klein et al. (1975) found that clinicians are most likely to use computer systems that give rapid feedback and help with record keeping. Slack et al. (1967) reported that clinicians find computer summaries very useful, because they relieve the clinician of an onerous chart-keeping task and free him or her for more reinforcing activities such as direct patient care. Quaak et al. (1986) found that computer-generated medical histories contained more complete information than did conventional histories and that clinicians were of the clear opinion that the computerized record was of most value before seeing the patient for the first time. The Voice DISC can produce a variety of reports—ranging from diagnostic checklists, through criterion and symptom scale reports, to printouts of questions and responses that occurred during the interview—within a few seconds of the end of an interview (Fisher et al. 1993b).

Psychometric Performance of the Voice DISC. The Voice DISC, an audio-CASI version of the Present State DISC, has been extensively used in school screenings and clinical facilities. Formal psychometric testing has been carried out in 400 subjects (delinquent youths) in residential care at Boys Town. These subjects were randomly allocated to one of four groups ($n=100$/group) who were interviewed on two occasions separated by a few days. Two groups received both methods of administration—the computerized self-report and conventional lay interviewer administration—in counterbalanced fashion (i.e., one group received computerized self-report followed by conventional lay interviewer administration and the other group received the opposite). Two other groups received the same method repeated twice to measure test-retest reliability. Data on the first 222 subjects from all four experimental groups are presented elsewhere (C.P. Lucas 2001); additional data are presented here on the test-retest component groups receiving the Present State DISC by human interviewer ($n=100$) and the Voice DISC by self-administration

($n=97$). The sample was 58% male; ethnicity was 61% Caucasian, 21% African American, 9% Hispanic, 3% Native American, 7% Mixed/Other, and 1% Unknown. The age range was 9–18 years (mean, 14.78). Initial estimates show that mean administration time for the Voice DISC was 65 minutes (approximately 30% that obtained by conventional lay administration). Acceptability was high, with over 70% of the adolescent subjects who expressed a preference preferring self-administration to conventional interviewer administration. Test-retest data (Table 3–4) showed some differences in the reliability of diagnoses between the self-administered and the interviewer-administered DISC, but these did not follow any specific pattern. Reliability (κ) statistics are presented only where the number of positive cases is five or greater at either time 1 or time 2. The mean κ value across all diagnoses for the Voice DISC mode of administration was 0.52, for the person-administered Present State DISC it was 0.47; this difference were not significant.

Validity of Computerized Self-Assessments

Of particular interest is the suggestion that people seem to prefer revealing some types of very personal information (e.g., gynecological details [Slack and Van Cura 1968], sexual abuse histories [Bagley and Genius 1991], and suicidal ideation [Greist et al. 1973]) to a computer rather than to a person. As well as being preferred by subjects, the computer also sometimes seems able to elicit more accurate reports of suicidal ideation and attempts than are elicited by clinicians (Beck et al. 1988; Levine et al. 1989). It has also been reported that alcoholics seeking treatment disclose greater levels of consumption of alcohol to a computer than to a person (R.W. Lucas et al. 1977).

Studies of the possibility of increased disclosure of adolescents' symptoms to computers have been very limited. C.P. Lucas (1990) found no differences in parental reports of "socially sensitive" symptoms in children and adolescents (including suicidal ideation) using lay interviewers or computer interviewing. A community survey (Stanton et al. 1993) of adolescent risk-taking behavior that used a computer (with a recorded voice) did

Table 3–4. Test-retest of the Voice DISC compared with human interviewing

	Voice DISC (self-administration)		Present State DISC (human interviewer)	
	κ	SE	κ	SE
Agoraphobia	0.64	0.15	0.31	0.01
Agoraphobia without panic	0.71	0.16	−0.02	0.01
Generalized anxiety disorder	0.48	0.22	—	—
Obsessive-compulsive disorder	0.13	0.16	0.49	0.16
Separation anxiety	0.55	0.10	0.35	0.13
Social phobia	0.29	0.18	−0.04	0.02
Specific phobia	0.16	0.17	0.43	0.17
Any tic disorder	0.42	0.16	0.19	0.19
Major depression	0.37	0.20	—	—
Conduct disorder	0.66	0.08	0.64	0.08
Oppositional defiant disorder	0.44	0.16	0.39	0.17
ADHD, any type	0.19	0.19	0.48	0.22
Alcohol abuse	0.73	0.10	0.49	0.13
Alcohol dependence	0.47	0.18	0.48	0.15
Marijuana abuse	0.66	0.12	0.59	0.13
Marijuana dependence	0.72	0.10	0.66	0.12
Nicotine dependence	0.66	0.09	0.50	0.12
Other substance dependence	0.64	0.16	0.65	0.19

Note. ADHD=attention-deficit/hyperactivity disorder.

show a tendency for greater-than-expected reports of drug and alcohol usage, criminality, and suicide attempts by adolescents. The significance of these findings must be qualified, however, by the fact that the research design failed to include a comparable control group. A recent study of adolescent sexual behavior, drug use, and violence (Turner et al. 1998) showed more striking results for the preferential reporting of socially sensitive material to computers. This study reported findings from 1,690 respondents ages 15–19 years in the 1995 National Survey of Adolescent Males who were questioned using either audio-CASI or questionnaire. The increased reports of adolescent male-male sex (5.5%) make estimates more compatible with adults' retrospective reports of such behavior when they were adolescents. Overall, the prevalence rates for adolescent drug use were twice as high as had been seen in previous surveys not using this mode of administration. However, little difference was seen in reporting of mild or moderate alcohol and marijuana use.

In the Boys Town study (C.P. Lucas 2001), using preliminary data, the effect of mode of administration (self-administered Voice DISC versus interviewer-administered Present State DISC) was studied. Significantly increased rates of reporting were found with the Voice DISC for separation anxiety disorder, social phobia, any tic disorder, major depressive disorder, and nicotine dependence. Similar increased reporting was seen for generalized anxiety disorder and conduct disorder, but these differences just failed to reach statistical significance ($P=0.06$). To test the hypothesis that certain socially sensitive symptoms would be reported with greater frequency, stem questions that were significantly different in frequency were examined. Of the 14 symptoms that differed in frequency, 12 of them had higher reporting rates with the Voice DISC than with the person-administered Present State DISC. Although some of these symptoms are socially sensitive (e.g., "More interested in sex than usual" and "Did things you later wished you hadn't done"), the major effect for mode of administration was seen in anxiety symptoms and diagnoses—problems that may be more embarrassing for delinquent and antisocial adolescents to disclose.

Impact of Computerized Assessment on Clinical Services

A small number of earlier studies addressed the question of whether a combination of a comprehensive automated assessment of symptomatology with a subsequent sensitive exploration of presenting complaints by a clinician might represent the optimal approach. However, all the studies had serious methodological shortcomings, principally very little power to reject the null hypothesis.

Williams et al. (1975) described the impact of using routine evaluation by computer on an adult psychiatric service. The computerized evaluations appeared to reduce lengths of inpatient stay and increase outpatient turnover. However, there was no control group, and changes in treatment practices or the types of patients being admitted may have been responsible for the changes observed. In a different study, clinicians who had an opportunity to review a patient's answers to a computer interview were thought to be able to do a more focused assessment of the patient's functioning and to follow up questions raised by the interview report (Farrell et al. 1987), although again this was not tested experimentally.

Yokley and Reuter (1989) used a self-completion questionnaire for parents of children attending child psychiatric outpatient clinics. These data were subsequently entered into a computer, and the therapists were provided with a diagnostic report utilizing DSM-III criteria. It was believed that the report enabled clinicians to come to a diagnosis earlier in the evaluation process, although this was not specifically tested in the design of the study. One of the main problems with this study was the need to transfer parental reports from paper questionnaires onto a mainframe computer before analysis could take place. This led to a delay before reports were available to the clinicians, the possible introduction of coding or transcribing errors, and the increased possibility of incomplete and spurious responses.

Finally, in a small-scale, uncontrolled study Sawyer and colleagues (1992) investigated the effect of providing clinicians with a report from a computer-assisted interview conducted before their clinical assessment of children referred to a mental health service. The results suggested that the availability of reports from computer-assisted interviews influenced the type of problems identified by clinicians and the services they recommended to manage the children's problems.

All of these previous reports were essentially uncontrolled naturalistic studies with little attempt to control for the experimenter effect (i.e., in which changes in practice are attributable to being observed) (Kintz et al. 1965) or to control for changes in referral or diagnostic practices that may have been due to secular changes (increased awareness or recognition of a particular disorder), responses to external events (e.g., disaster-related symptoms), or seasonally mediated changes in identification (e.g., associated with the school calendar). Despite these limitations, they do appear to show that computer-generated reports are of some value to clinicians and that diagnostic and other clinical behavior may change as a result of the availability of such information and systems.

However, there may be some potential drawbacks that could arise from the introduction of standardized systems of assessment into clinical services. These may affect certain types of settings or types of clinicians differentially (Leaper et al. 1972). For example, the extra information may confuse clinicians or lead them to focus too greatly on certain areas (e.g., symptoms) to the detriment of other relevant foci (e.g., context). Also, patients or parents may find the assessments boring or intrusive and thus drop out more frequently during evaluation. There is an urgent need, therefore, for research to scientifically address the impact of the introduction and use of such standardized assessment procedures on clinical services, using appropriate controls and design safeguards.

One such study has been carried out, and preliminary data on clients and clinicians have been presented (Mullen et al. 1999). These analyses included 21 clinicians and 95 children and youths from four outpatient child psychiatric clinics in the New York metropolitan area where routine evaluation with the lay interviewer–administered C-DISC was implemented for new patients immediately before their first assessment visit. Data are compared to a control, baseline period in the clinic when subjects and clinicians merely completed checklists measuring satisfaction with the assessment procedures. The sample included 45 (47.4%) females and 50 (52.6%) males. The age distribution ranged from 9 to 17 years, with a modal age of 10 and a median of 12. Of the 95 youths, 37 (38.9%) were African American or Black, 26 (27.3%) were Latino or Latina, 18 (18.9%) were white, six (6.3%) were biracial or of mixed race or ethnicity, and two (2.1%) were classified as of another racial or ethnic group.

Initial findings demonstrated that more than 85% of the clinicians found the C-DISC to have been "helpful" in at least one of their cases. For some, the C-DISC protocol was found to be helpful in even more of their cases, because in the entire sample approximately two-fifths of the patients reportedly benefited from the C-DISC information. There was no evidence that the C-DISC was viewed as overly intrusive or simply redundant. The value of the C-DISC information to the clinician was demonstrated by the facts that the majority of clinicians reported that the C-DISC had changed their evaluations in at least one of their cases and that in about one-fifth of the cases the clinicians said that the C-DISC report had changed their evaluations.

Concerns regarding possible negative effects of the introduction into clinical practice of a computerized, highly structured diagnostic protocol such as the C-DISC were not supported in the majority of cases in this study. Approximately one-half of the clinicians reported that the C-DISC never made an interview with a child, youth, or caretaker more difficult. In fact, in approximately three-quarters of the child and youth interviews and four-fifths of the caretaker interviews the C-DISC did not make the intake interviews more difficult. Similarly, most clinicians reported that the C-DISC had never visibly upset a child, youth, or caretaker whom they saw for intake interviews; and when asked, most children, youths, and caretakers in the study did not report being upset by the C-DISC.

Parent and youth reports of feeling understood and of being able to discuss concerns were examined, contrasting the two assessment conditions (baseline and after introduction of the C-DISC). Two significant effects were found that favored the C-DISC condition: 1) according to the clinicians' assessment, the caretakers were more fully able to discuss their concerns after administration of the C-DISC; and 2) the caretakers' satisfaction with the intake session increased after introduction of the C-DISC.

These findings suggest that in most cases the benefits attributed by the clinicians to the C-DISC information were not offset by risks to patients or caretakers.

Summary

The difficult process of establishing a psychiatric diagnosis is compounded by the heterogeneous training of mental health clinicians that may focus on features such as family dynamics or specific behaviors at the expense of a phenomenological diagnosis.

Standardized diagnostic interviews such as the inexpensively administered C-DISC could potentially alleviate such resulting clinical problems as inaccurate diagnosis and inappropriate treatment or the underidentification of diagnoses for which specific treatments are available.

Economic advantages could include a reduction in the amount of time taken to come to a complete assessment and a reduction in wasted treatment time brought about by the wrong diagnosis.

The introduction of routine standardized assessments could also assist in the assurance of quality control. The availability of objective and quantifiable baseline measures could provide a basis for evaluating treatment effects and could lead to the establishment of expert systems that will allow auditors to determine the appropriateness of a given intervention.

The accuracy of assessments made with structured interviews is comparable to the accuracy of those made by a clinician. Because of their accuracy—in addition to their significant cost advantages, the comprehensive nature of the diagnostic assessment afforded by the standardized approach, and the opportunities for improved quality control—structured interviews open exciting new possibilities for clinical, research, and preventive activities.

References

Achenbach TM, Edelbrock CS: Manual for the Child Behavior Checklist and Revised Child Behavior Profile. Burlington, VT, Department of Psychiatry, University of Vermont, 1983

Achenbach TM, Edelbrock CS: Manual for the Child Behavior Checklist: Youth Self Report. Burlington, VT, Department of Psychiatry, University of Vermont, 1987

Achenbach TM, Conners CK, Quay HC: The ACQ Behavior Checklist. Burlington, VT, Department of Psychiatry, University of Vermont, 1993

American Psychiatric Association: Diagnostic and Statistical Manual of Mental Disorders, 3rd Edition. Washington, DC, American Psychiatric Association, 1980

American Psychiatric Association: Diagnostic and Statistical Manual of Mental Disorders, 3rd Edition, Revised. Washington, DC, American Psychiatric Association, 1987

American Psychiatric Association: Diagnostic and Statistical Manual of Mental Disorders, 4th Edition. Washington, DC, American Psychiatric Association, 1994

American Psychiatric Association: Diagnostic and Statistical Manual of Mental Disorders, 4th Edition, Text Revision. Washington, DC, American Psychiatric Association, 2000

Angold A, Costello EJ: A test-retest reliability study of child-reported psychiatric symptoms and diagnoses using the Child and Adolescent Psychiatric Assessment (CAPA-C). Psychol Med 25:755–762, 1995

Angold A, Prendergast M, Cox A, et al: The Child and Adolescent Psychiatric Assessment (CAPA). Psychol Med 25:739–753, 1995

Anthony JC, Folstein M, Romanoski AJ, et al: Comparison of the lay Diagnostic Interview Schedule and a standardized psychiatric diagnosis: experience in Eastern Baltimore. Arch Gen Psychiatry 42:667–675, 1985

Bagley C, Genius M: Psychology of computer use: XX. Sexual abuse recalled: evaluation of a computerized questionnaire in a population of young adult males. Percept Mot Skills 72:287–288, 1991

Beck AT, Steer RA, Ranieri WF: Scale for suicidal ideation: psychometric properties of a self report version. J Clin Psychol 44:499–505, 1988

Berg I, Lucas CP, McGuire R: Measurement of behaviour difficulties in children using standard scales administered to mothers by computer: reliability and validity. Eur Child Adolesc Psychiatry 1:14–23, 1992

Bradburn NM, Sudman S: Improving Interview Method and Questionnaire Design. San Francisco, CA, Jossey-Bass, 1979

Burgoyne RW: The structured interview—an aid to compiling a clear and concise data base. Int J Ment Health 6:37–48, 1977

Coddington RD, King TL: Automated history taking in child psychiatry. Am J Psychiatry 129:276–282, 1972

Cohen J: A coefficient of agreement for nominal scales. Educ Psychol Meas 20:37–46, 1960

Costello AJ, Edelbrock C, Dulcan MK et al: Report on the NIMH Diagnostic Interview Schedule for Children (DISC). Washington, DC, National Institute of Mental Health, 1984

Edelbrock C, Costello A, Dulcan MK, et al: Age differences in the reliability of the psychiatric interview of the child. Child Dev 56:265–275, 1985

Elstein AS, Kagan N, Shulman LS, et al: Methods and theory in the study of medical inquiry. J Med Educ 47:85–92, 1972

Erdman HP, Klein MH, Greist JH: Direct patient computer interviewing. J Consult Clin Psychol 53:760–773, 1985

Fallon T, Schwab-Stone M: Determinants of reliability in psychiatric surveys of children aged 6–12. J Child Psychol Psychiatry 35:1391–1408, 1994

Farrell AD, Camplair PS, McCullough L: Identification of target complaints by computer interview: evaluation of the computerized assessment system for psychotherapy evaluation and research. J Consult Clin Psychol 55:691–700, 1987

Fisher P, Shaffer D, Piacentini JC, et al: Sensitivity of the Diagnostic Interview Schedule for Children, 2nd edition (DISC 2.1) for specific diagnoses of children and adolescents. J Am Acad Child Adolesc Psychiatry 32:666–673, 1993a

Fisher P, Blouin A, Shaffer D: The C-DISC: A computerized version of the NIMH Diagnostic Interview Schedule for Children, Version 2.3. Poster presentation at International Society for Research in Child and Adolescent Psychopathology, Santa Fe, NM, June 1993b

Gauron EF, Dickinson JK: Diagnostic decision making in psychiatry, II: Diagnostic styles. Arch Gen Psychiatry 14:233–237, 1966a

Gauron EF, Dickinson JK: Diagnostic decision making in psychiatry, I: Information usage. Arch Gen Psychiatry 14:225–232, 1966b

Graham P, Rutter M: The reliability and validity of the psychiatric assessment of the child: II. Interview with the parent. Br J Psychiatry 114:581–592, 1968

Greist JH, Gustafson DH, Stauss FF, et al: A computer interview for suicide risk prediction. Am J Psychiatry 130:1327–1332, 1973

Herjanic B, Reich W: Development of a structured psychiatric interview for children: agreement between child and parent on individual symptoms. J Abnorm Child Psychol 10:307–324, 1982

Jensen P, Roper M, Fisher P, et al: Test-retest reliability of the Diagnostic Interview Schedule for Children (Version 2.1): parent, child, and combined algorithms. Arch Gen Psychiatry 52:61–71, 1995

Kendell RE: Psychiatric diagnoses: a study of how they are made. Br J Psychiatry 122:437–445, 1973

Kendell RE: Diagnosis as a practical decision-making process, in The Role of Diagnosis in Psychiatry. Oxford, Blackwell, 1975, pp 49–59

Kintz BL, Delprato DJ, Mettee DR, et al: The experimenter effect. Psychol Bull 63:223–232, 1965

Klein MH, Greist JH, Van Cura LJ: Computers and psychiatry: promises to keep. Arch Gen Psychiatry 32:837–843, 1975

Lahey BB, Flagg EW, Bird HR, et al: The NIMH Methods for the Epidemiology of Child and Adolescent Mental Disorders (MECA) Study: background and methodology. J Am Acad Child Adolesc Psychiatry 35:855–864, 1996

Leaper DJ, Horrocks JC, Staniland JR, et al: Computer-assisted diagnosis of abdominal pain using "estimates" provided by clinicians. Br Med J 4:350–354, 1972

Levine S, Ancill RJ, Roberts AP: Assessment of suicide risk by computer-delivered self-rating questionnaire: preliminary findings. Acta Psychiatr Scand 80:216–220, 1989

Lucas CP: Computerised administration of behavioral rating scales: a comparative study. Unpublished master's thesis, Leeds University, Leeds, U.K., 1990

Lucas CP: The order effect: reflections on the validity of multiple test presentations. Psychol Med 22:197–202, 1992

Lucas CP: Automated assessment of symptoms and diagnoses: theory and practice. Workshop presentation at the 48th annual meeting of the American Academy of Child and Adolescent Psychiatry, Honolulu, HI, October 2001

Lucas CP, Fisher P, Shaffer D: NIMH Diagnostic Interview Schedule for Children—Present State Version. Unpublished interview schedule. New York, Department of Child Psychiatry, Columbia University, 1997

Lucas CP, Fisher P, Piacentini J, et al: Features of interview questions associated with attenuation of symptom reports. J Abnorm Child Psychol 27:429–437, 1999

Lucas RW, Mullin PJ, Luna CBX, et al: Psychiatrists and a computer as interrogators of patients with alcohol-related illnesses: a comparison. Br J Psychiatry 131:160–167, 1977

Mullen E: Using assessment instruments in social work practice. Paper presented at the 2nd annual meeting of the International Inter-Centre Network for Evaluation of Social Work Practice: Researcher-Practitioner Partnerships and Research Implementation, Stockholm, 1999

Piacentini JC, Shaffer D, Fisher P, et al: The Diagnostic Interview Schedule for Children-Revised version (DISC-R): III. Concurrent criterion validity. J Am Acad Child Adolesc Psychiatry 32:658–665, 1993

Puig-Antich J, Chambers W: The Schedule for Affective Disorders and Schizophrenia for School-Aged Children. Unpublished interview schedule. New York, New York State Psychiatric Institute, 1978

Quaak MJ, Westerman RF, Schouten JA, et al: Appraisal of computerized medical histories: comparisons between computerized and conventional records. Comput Biomed Res 19:551–564, 1986

Roberts RE, Solovitz BL, Chen YW, et al: Retest stability of DSM-III-R diagnoses among adolescents using the Diagnostic Interview Schedule for Children (DISC-2.1C). J Abnorm Child Psychol 24:349–361, 1996

Sawyer MG, Sarris A, Baghurst P: The use of a computer-assisted interview to administer the Child Behavior Checklist in a child psychiatry service. J Am Acad Child Adolesc Psychiatry 30:674–681, 1991

Sawyer MG, Sarris A, Baghurst P: The effect of computer-assisted interviewing on the clinical assessment of children. Aust N Z J Psychiatry 26:223–231, 1992

Schwab-Stone M, Fisher P, Piacentini JC, et al: The Diagnostic Interview Schedule for Children-Revised Version (DISC-R): II. Test-retest reliability. J Am Acad Child Adolesc Psychiatry 32:651–657, 1993

Schwab-Stone ME, Shaffer D, Dulcan MK, et al: Criterion validity of the NIMH Diagnostic Interview Schedule for Children (DISC-2.3). J Am Acad Child Adolesc Psychiatry 35:878–888, 1996

Setterberg S, Ernst M, Rao U, et al: Child psychiatrists' views of DSM-III-R: a survey of usage and opinions. J Am Acad Child Adolesc Psychiatry 30:652–658, 1991

Shaffer D, Schwab-Stone M, Fisher P, et al: The Diagnostic Interview Schedule for Children-Revised Version (DISC-R): I. Preparation, field testing, inter-rater reliability, and acceptability. J Am Acad Child Adolesc Psychiatry 32:643–650, 1993

Shaffer D, Fisher P, Dulcan MK, et al: The NIMH Diagnostic Interview Schedule for Children (DISC-2.3): description, acceptability, prevalence, and relationship to global measures of impairment, and characteristics of measures of onset and impairment. J Am Acad Child Adolesc Psychiatry 35:865–877, 1996

Shaffer D, Fisher P, Lucas C, et al: NIMH Diagnostic Interview Schedule for Children, Version IV (NIMH DISC-IV): description, differences from previous versions, and reliability of some common diagnoses. J Am Acad Child Adolesc Psychiatry 39:28–38, 2000

Shrout PE, Fleiss JL: Intra-class correlations: uses in assessing rater reliability. Psychol Bull 2:420–428, 1979

Simon RJ, Gurland BJ, Fleiss JL, et al: Impact of a patient history interview on psychiatric diagnosis. Arch Gen Psychiatry 24:437–440, 1971

Slack WV, Van Cura LJ: Patient reactions to computer-based medical interviewing. Comput Biomed Res 1:527–531, 1968

Slack WV, Peckham BM, Van Cura LJ, et al: A computer-based physical examination system. JAMA 200:136–140, 1967

Stanton B, Romer D, Ricardo I, et al: Early initiation of sex and its lack of association with risk behaviors among adolescent African-Americans. Pediatrics 92:13–19, 1993

Turner CF, Ku L, Rogers SM, et al: Adolescent sexual behavior, drug use, and violence: increased reporting with computer survey technology. Science 280:867–873, 1998

Williams TA, Johnson JH, Bliss EL: A computer-assisted psychiatric assessment unit. Am J Psychiatry 132:1074–1076, 1975

Wing JK, Cooper JE, Sartorious N: The Measurement and Classification of Psychiatric Symptoms. London, Cambridge University Press, 1974

World Health Organization: International Classification of Diseases, 10th Edition. Geneva, World Health Organization, 1993

Yokley JM, Reuter JM: The computer assisted child diagnostic system: a research and development project. Comput Human Behav 5:277–295, 1989

Chapter 4

Risk Factors for Suicidal Behavior

The Utility and Limitations of Research Instruments

Maria A. Oquendo, M.D.
Batsheva Halberstam, B.A.
J. John Mann, M.D.

There are about 30,000 suicides per year in the United States, making it the 11th leading cause of death in the country (National Center for Injury Prevention and Control 2002). Somewhere from 10 to 20 times that number attempt suicide and survive. Yet although identification of those at risk for suicidal behavior could prevent the significant morbidity and mortality associated with these behaviors, this goal remains elusive. Roy (1982) found that of 75 outpatients who had committed suicide, 58% had seen a psychiatrist the week before their death. One study (Isacsson et al. 1992) conducted in Sweden revealed that in the 3 months before suicide, about half of the subjects had received medical attention. In San Diego, California, two-thirds of the suicide victims consulted a physician in the 90 days before their suicide. Isometsa et al. (1994) found that in Finland, two-thirds of patients with a history of major depressive disorder at the time of suicide had received psychiatric treatment during their last year of life. Thus, studies suggest that recognition and identification of immi-

Supported by Conte Center for the Study of the Neurobiology of Suicidal Behavior and NIMH grant MH59710.

nent suicide victims is poor. In this chapter, we provide definitions for different types of suicidal behavior. We also include a brief description of some of the clinical and neurobiological risk factors for suicidal behavior that have been identified in the literature. Following a brief description of clinical and research approaches to assessment of suicide risk, examples of research scales that have been proposed as being useful in risk assessment are described and the literature regarding their utility is discussed.

Definitions of Suicidal Behavior

Significant obstacles have hampered the accurate prediction of risk for suicide. Most salient is the problem of defining suicidal behavior and a lack of uniform nomenclature or classification for suicidal behavior. For example, a particular behavior may be labeled a "suicide attempt," a "suicidal gesture," or a "manipulative suicide attempt," depending solely on the clinical or research setting (O'Carroll et al. 1996). Because of this problem, the National Institute of Mental Health (2002), as well as individual researchers (Beck et al. 1973; Maris et al. 1992), have proposed classification systems for suicidal behavior. However, none of these classification schemes are widely accepted, and suicidal behavior is still classified using a variety of schemata.

In 1972, the Center for Studies of Suicide Prevention at the National Institute of Mental Health proposed three categories of suicidal behavior: completed suicide, attempted suicide, and suicidal ideas (Beck et al. 1975a, 1979). These definitions have more recently been refined by O'Carroll et al. (1996). Adjusting the definition of suicide attempts or completion to a more general term, *suicide-related behavior*, two subcategories are described: instrumental behavior and suicidal acts. Instrumental behavior is self-injurious behavior that is *not* intended to be lethal but has some other purpose, such as help seeking. Instrumental behavior can have one of three outcomes—no injury, injury, or death. It is the lack of intent to die that differentiates instrumental behavior from suicidal acts. The other subcategory of suicide-related behavior is suicidal acts. These are self-injurious acts committed by an individual with either explicit or implicit intent to die. If the outcome of the suicidal act is death, it is called a completed suicide. If the individual survives the suicidal act either with or without injury, it is a suicide attempt. This distinguishing feature between suicide attempt and instrumental behavior—namely, the intent of the individual—requires assessment in potentially suicidal patients. One difficulty with the subdivision by O'Carroll et al. (1996) is that it is not uncommon for patients to admit to suicidal intent when first seen in the emergency room and then to strenuously deny any intent to die after admission to the hospital. This may be due to the psychological mechanism of denial, or it may be a deliberate endeavor on the patient's part to convince the staff to discharge him or her sooner. The report by the Institute of Medicine in 2002 took the position that a suicide attempt is an act of self-harm with some intent to end one's life, and that intent could be inferred from the lethality of the act or from statements made by the individual at the time of the act or later (Goldsmith et al. 2002). Retraction of an earlier statement is not accepted. The most serious statement of intent is the measure of intent. Suicidal intent is defined as the seriousness or intensity of the patient's wish to terminate his or her life (Beck et al. 1974a). Inquiry about the purpose of the attempt, the patient's suicidal planning, perception of the outcome in terms of fatality, steps to prevent discovery of the suicide plan before enough time is elapsed to ensure success of the method, arrangements for death such as preparing a will or purchasing life insurance, gives information about the degree of suicidal intent.

Suicidal ideation encompasses thoughts about the desire and method for committing suicide (Beck et al. 1988). It has various dimensions, including the presence of a current plan for killing oneself and the availability of means to do so. Suicidal ideation may be of varying intensity, ranging from occasional fleeting thoughts to intrusive persistent ruminations about one's own death. In addition, patients often can identify reasons that they find compelling for or against killing themselves. Assessment of ideation for the purpose of short-term assessment of risk involves scoring the most serious suicidal ideation in the last few days.

These factors are important aspects of suicide risk assessment. Knowledge regarding the presence of some or all of these behaviors in a patient's history will enhance the clinician's ability to make a judgment about the person's risk of acting on suicidal thoughts. In the event that the individual has made a recent suicide attempt, the method employed and the seriousness of the injury sustained should be recorded because the lethality of past suicidal behavior may be related to the risk for future suicide. This also provides an indication of method preference and allows steps to deny access to the same method.

Clinical Risk Factors for Suicidal Behavior

We have proposed a stress-diathesis model for suicidal behavior (Mann et al. 1999) that posits that for suicidal behavior to occur there must be a precipitant or trigger (stress) as well as a preexisting vulnerability to suicidal behavior (diathesis). Examples of factors that may be stressors or triggers that can contribute to the timing of suicidal acts include acute episodes of psychiatric disorders, of which the most common is major depressive disorder; a psychosocial crisis involving some kind of loss or anticipated adverse outcome; acute intoxication with substances that may disinhibit (such as alcohol or benzodiazepines) or that may alter mood (such as LSD); and suicide contagion. Clinical factors influencing the diathesis include impulsivity (for example, a history of impulsive aggressive behavior), a tendency for pessimism, hopelessness, perceiving fewer reasons for living, and chronic substance abuse. The impulsivity may be part of a personality disorder such as borderline or antisocial personality disorder. Certain physical illnesses, especially those affecting the brain, may enhance the development of depression or impulsivity. A reported childhood history of abuse is also associated with a higher rate of mood disorders and suicidal behavior in adulthood, and we have reported that it is associated with a higher level of impulsivity (Brodsky et al. 2001). A chronic lack of social support may be considered a part of the diathesis. A history of suicide attempts in the past is an important indicator of the presence of this diathesis. In fact, we have recently shown that for each suicide attempt in a patient's history, the risk of another attempt during a 2-year follow-up period increases by 30% (Oquendo et al. 2002). The presence of one or more of these risk factors affecting the diathesis should heighten the monitoring of the patient's exposure to stressors, because these are potential opportunities to prevent the stressor from precipitating suicidal acts. In addition to assessment of these clinical risk factors, elements of the patient's current mental status—such as the presence of suicidal ideation, indications of suicidal intent, lethality of the contemplated method, the individual's familiarity with the lethality of his or her method, and access to the lethal method decided on—contribute to the clinical formulation of suicide risk. Given all these precautions, the most determined patient will sometimes deny all suicidal ideation or intent to deliberately mislead the clinician and thereby avoid being thwarted in his or her efforts to commit suicide.

Neurobiological Factors in the Assessment of Suicidal Behavior

Neurobiological predictors—many of them related to serotinergic functioning—have been studied to enhance identification of individuals at risk for eventual suicide (for comprehensive reviews see Kamali et al. 2001 and Oquendo and Mann 1999). For example, studies of cerebrospinal fluid (CSF) have revealed that compared with psychiatric control subjects, lower levels of 5-hydroxyindoleacetic acid (5-HIAA) are found in patients who made previous suicide attempts and in those who eventually made an attempt or completed suicide (Asberg and Traskman 1981; Kamali et al. 2001; Nordstrom et al. 1994; Traskman et al. 1981). Furthermore, lower CSF levels of 5-HIAA have been found in suicide attempters with major depressive disorder, personality disorders, and schizophrenia (Oquendo and Mann 2000), suggesting that this association with suicidal behavior holds true across diagnostic categories. The CSF level of 5-HIAA is lower in those who made high-lethality suicide attempts compared with those who made low-lethality attempts (Mann and Malone 1997), indicating that seriousness of suicidal behavior makes a difference. Similarly, there is also substantial evidence suggesting that CSF 5-HIAA levels are related to impulsivity and aggressive behavior. Lower CSF levels of 5-HIAA are associated with serious impulsive aggression, and the level is lower in proportion to the severity of lifetime aggression (Linnoila et al. 1983; Virkkunen et al. 1994); these results were confirmed in aggressive nonattempter compared with nonaggressive nonattempters with psychiatric disorders (Stanley et al. 2000). Together with our finding that suicide attempters with major depressive disorder have higher levels of aggression and impulsivity than nonattempters (Mann et al. 1999), these data suggest that lower serotinergic functioning is associated with both aggression and an increased risk for suicidal behavior, and these two behaviors are in turn associated with each other (Oquendo and Mann 1999). Cutoff points to categorize patients' serotinergic function as high or low are not available. However, obtaining an aggression history in addition to a suicide attempt history may enhance the clinician's assessment of suicide risk.

Genetic studies have revealed a higher concordance rate of suicide in monozygotic twins than in dizygotic twins (Roy et al. 1995). The Copenhagen Adoption study (Schulsinger and Knop 1977) found that, independent of the transmission of a major psychiatric disorder, adoptees who committed suicide had a sixfold higher rate of suicide in their biological relatives than matched adoptees who had not committed suicide. None of the adopting relatives committed suicide. Furthermore, Statham et al. (1998) found that a history of suicide attempt or suicidal thoughts predicts the same phenomena in monozygotic twins but not in dizygotic twins. Similarly, in a comparison of offspring of depressed suicide attempters to offspring of depressed individuals with no prior history of suicidal acts, we recently found that having a parent with a history of suicidal behavior elevated the risk for suicidal acts in the offspring sixfold (Brent et al. 2002). These studies on the heritability of suicidal behavior strongly support the idea that suicidal behavior runs in families. Whether this heritability is genetic, environmental, or both still requires clarification. Regardless, inquiry about a family history of suicidal acts must be part of an evaluation of suicide risk.

Clinical Assessment of Suicide Risk

Many clinicians employ the no-harm contract in their assessment of and interaction with potentially suicidal patients. The contract is a verbal or written agreement in which the patient affirms that he or she will not kill himself or herself for a specific period of time (Miller et al. 1998). Although the utility of the no-harm contract for suicide prevention has not been determined, the contract can be used as a risk assessment tool (Stanford et al. 1994). Observation of the patient's response when asked to participate in a no-harm contract can provide clues to the patient's commitment not to act on suicidal ideation. The contract also provides a structure for establishing a plan, together with the patient, about what the patient should do if the suicidal ideation becomes more severe or if the patient feels unable to control suicidal impulses. Nonetheless, the clinician must recognize the limitations of the no-harm contract and the fact that it does not guarantee safety even in the case that the patient agrees to it.

The best single clinical predictor of a future suicide attempt is a previous suicide attempt (Malone et al. 1995; Steer et al. 1988). Therefore, the clinical evaluation of suicide risk must include a history of the number and medical severity of suicide attempts. The clinician establishes the degree of suicide intent during the past attempts and also makes an assessment of suicidal ideation at those times. That information can assist the clinician in evaluating the risk that current suicidal ideation and suicidal intent pose for the particular patient. It allows the clinician to take into account the fact that patients vary in their threshold for acting on suicidal thoughts. As mentioned above under "Clinical Risk Factors for Suicidal Behavior," assessment of the presence of borderline personality disorder, family history of suicidal behavior, personal history of aggression, and other clinical factors can also assist in establishing risk. Protective factors such as specific reasons for not acting on suicidal ideation can provide evidence for decreased risk.

Clinicians face several obstacles when assessing suicide risk (Chiles and Strosahl 1995). They often have only a brief time to determine the intensity of an individual's suicide risk and to establish whether the patient might be attempting suicide that day or the next. Furthermore, current approaches to the assessment of risk cannot offer reasonable estimates of the length of time between the assessment point and any attempt that may occur subsequently. Level of risk may change over time, depending on variations in the patient's psychiatric condition or life events. Indeed, risk may improve or be exacerbated by external circumstances even within a short period of time (Pallis et al. 1984). Yet the clinician must intervene if he or she suspects imminent risk, despite the fact that it is often impossible to be certain of the patient's imminent risk for making a suicide attempt. Moreover, unnecessary hospitalization may also bring complications. Costs to the patient are often both emotional and financial. These compelling reasons have led researchers to try to develop scales that can accurately predict risk of suicide.

Research Assessment of Suicide Risk

Studies attempting to predict eventual suicide prospectively have yet to yield an approach with good sensitivity and specificity. Standard psychological tests—such as the Minnesota Multiphasic Personality Inventory, the Thematic Apperception Test, and the Rorschach test—generally do not identify those at risk for suicidal acts and are not useful predictors (Beck et al. 1979). Previous studies have shown very low rates of sensitivity, demonstrating that suicides are difficult to predict with currently identified risk factors or available scales (Beck et al. 1999; Pokorny 1993) For example, in 1993, Pokorny reported on a prospective study in which 4,800 psychiatric inpatients were observed for 10 years. He attempted to predict eventual suicide completion based on a combination of factors such as history of suicide attempts, marital status, and psychiatric diagnosis. He was able to predict only 9 of 73 suicides, with a sensitivity of 29% and a specificity of 99%. Studies such as Pokorny's have shown that although certain research instruments are able to recognize increased risk over time, they do not necessarily identify imminent risk.

In a similar study, Beck et al. (1999) observed 3,701 outpatients between 1975 and 1994. Clinicians administered the Scale for Suicide Ideation to assess both current ideation and ideation at its worst point in the patient's life. Patients were classified as either lower risk or higher risk based on cutoff scores. For current suicidal ideation, a score of 0–1 was classified as lower risk, and 2–38 was classified as higher risk. For ideation at its worst point in life, a score of 0–15 was considered lower risk, whereas a score of 16–38 was higher risk. Patients who were in the higher-risk category as measured by the scale for ideation at its worst point were 14 times more likely to commit suicide than those in the lower-risk category. For current ideation, patients who were in the higher-risk category were found to be six times more likely to commit suicide than those in the lower-risk category. This suggests that to determine lifetime risk for suicidal behavior, both current and worst ideation should be assessed, especially because the patient may not be experiencing his or her worst ideation at time of the interview. However, this scale was used to predict lifetime risk rather than imminent risk, which is clearly a more pressing concern in the clinical situation. Thus, research scales have utility in studying large groups of subjects about lifetime risk but do not offer specific enough information to be reliable in assessment of imminent suicide risk in individuals.

Research Versus Clinical Assessments of Suicide Risk

Research assessments are reported to differ from the clinical information recorded in hospital charts, with the patient's risk of suicide and history of suicide attempts usually being underestimated in clinical interviews. In the only study we could identify comparing research and clinical assessment of suicide risk, Malone et al. (1995) found that clinical assessments failed to record a previous suicide attempt in 24% of cases at admission and 28% of cases at discharge. In addition, the discharge summary did not document suicidal ideation or planning at the time of admission for the current hospitalization in 38% of patients. Therefore, suicidal behavior recorded in the clinical discharge summary was significantly less accurate than that recorded on the research assessments, which resulted in the loss of critical clinical information when the patient was referred for follow-up treatment after hospitalization. This may contribute to the already difficult task of identifying patients who will attempt or complete suicide and suggests that patient interviews focused on current suicidal risk may be improved through the use of a semistructured suicide interview (Malone et al. 1995).

Research Tools in the Assessment of Suicide Risk

We present some examples of instruments available to assess different aspects of suicidal behavior. As is the case in general, most of the instruments discussed focus on the evaluation of risk factors for suicidal acts. We also include a research scale that measures protective factors.

Columbia Suicide History Form

Research has shown that the best predictor of a future suicide attempt is a previous suicide attempt (Malone et al. 1995; Steer et al. 1988). The Columbia Suicide History Form (Appendix 4–1) is a semistructured instrument devised by our group (in New York and Pittsburgh) that asks information about lifetime suicide attempts, including the method, lethality, precipitant, and surrounding circumstances of the attempts (Oquendo et al. 1999).

Defining Suicidal Acts

The Columbia Suicide History Form distinguishes between actual, ambiguous, interrupted, and aborted attempts. An actual suicide attempt is defined as a self-injurious act committed with at least some intent to die, which does not have to be explicit. For example, if the attempter denies intent but thought his or her attempt would be lethal, the clinician can infer intent through the individual's method.

An interrupted attempt occurs when the attempter is interrupted and is prevented by outside circumstances from beginning the self-injurious behavior. Interrupted attempters are reported to be three times more likely to eventually commit suicide than uninterrupted attempters (Steer et al. 1988). Attempters who eventually completed a suicide attempt—those who, in a sense, learned their lesson from the interrupted attempt and took more precautions against being discovered—chose more isolated places or chose times when discovery was not likely.

An aborted attempt occurs when the individual begins the suicidal act but stops himself or herself before any self-destructive behavior has been completed. For example, the individual amasses enough pills to take in a lethal overdose, decides on a time and place to kill herself or himself, makes preparations to carry out the attempt, and at the last minute decides not to act (Marzuk et al. 1997). Although few studies have focused on this type of behavior, these subjects have been shown to be at risk for eventual attempts. Marzuk (1997) studied 733 patients, of whom 213 (29%) had made at least one aborted attempt. Subjects who had made an aborted attempt were also more likely to have made an actual attempt in the past. Aborted attempts may serve as a kind of rehearsal for the actual attempt. It is possible that an aborted attempt can be a predictor of an actual attempt; however, given the high lethality potential of some of the observed aborted attempts, prospective studies are necessary to confirm this hypothesis. A critical aspect of defining an aborted attempt is that it is not solely that the person had detailed suicidal ideation with a plan and availability of the contemplated method. Rather, the person must also report taking actual steps toward initiating a suicidal act, thus being in imminent danger of acting before deciding against it. In the previous example, the person may have gone to a remote location with the pills and poured the pills, but immediately before putting the pills in his or her mouth had a change of heart.

Finally, an ambiguous attempt is defined as a suicidal act that appears to have been carried out with intent to die, but the attempter denies intent and the clinician cannot infer it. This category of ambiguous attempt is used very rarely. For example, a patient may be adamant that the intent of an overdose was solely to sleep, yet reports taking 20 sleeping pills at one time. Most individuals would recognize this as an excessive number of pills, and an act that could potentially be lethal. Yet the overdose victim denies intent. The clinician may remain concerned about this patient's suicide potential and categorize this act as an ambiguous attempt.

Detailing the Circumstances Surrounding Each Suicide Attempt

The Columbia Suicide History Form records as many attempts as the individual has made in his or her lifetime. The suicide attempter is asked to give a narrative of each attempt. For each suicide attempt, the clinician establishes the date, precipitant, method, and lethality and identifies the first attempt, the most lethal attempt, and the most recent attempt.

The attempter is asked the date of each suicide attempt. If he or she is not able to specify the date of the attempt, an estimate of the date is recorded as indicated in the "Calculating Imprecision" section of the form. (See Appendix 4–1 for directions for calculations.)

The clinician assesses the precipitant, or trigger, of each attempt. The first seven categories for precipitant are based on the St. Paul-Ramsey Life Experience Scale and the DSM-IV-TR Axis IV categories (American Psychiatric Association 2000) (conjugal, other interpersonal, occupational, living situation, health, other, cannot be assessed). Two more categories, sexual abuse and physical abuse, were added when our team discovered they were frequent precipitants. These had previously been coded as "other interpersonal," "living situation," or "other." There is an additional space for a secondary trigger, if indicated.

The lethality of each attempt is calculated based on Beck's Lethality Rating Scale (Beck et al. 1975a) (see "Medical Lethality" below).

The Columbia Suicide History Form has demonstrated good reliability, and in our hands it shows an interrater reliability coefficient of 0.97. Because it accurately records an individual's history of suicide attempts and their number and lethality, this tool may facilitate identification of suicide risk.

Scale for Suicide Ideation

Suicidal ideation is the presence of thoughts or current plans to commit suicide. The severity of suicidal ideation is an indicator of an individual's risk of attempting suicide (Mann et al. 1999). The Scale for Suicide Ideation is a reliable method for measuring an individual's severity of suicidal ideation (Beck et al. 1988). The Scale for Suicide Ideation is designed to quantify the intensity of current, conscious suicidal ideas and focuses on the pervasiveness and characteristics of the ideation. In addition, the scale measures suicidal communications expressed in overt behavior or those that are verbalized. Questions on the scale were originally selected to reflect the range of suicidal preoccupations most frequently observed in patients (Beck et al. 1979). Each question on the scale assesses the intensity of the individual's suicidal thoughts as well as his or her attitude toward them. Unlike the Suicide Intent Scale (see below), the Scale for Suicide Ideation can be completed for nonattempters as well as attempters (Beck et al. 1975b). It is a 19-item instrument on which the clinician rates the severity of a patient's suicidal thoughts and plans on a 3-point scale (0–2). Ratings add up to a total score, from 0 to 38. A rating that is positive for suicidal ideation means that further clinical intervention is necessary.

Beck et al. (1990) found that psychiatric inpatients who eventually completed suicide did not score higher in suicidal ideation than patients who did not commit suicide. However, when patients were asked about suicidal ideation at its worst point in their lives, those who had higher scores were 14 times more likely to commit suicide than those with lower scores. Those who scored higher on current suicidal ideation were about six times more likely to commit suicide than those with lower scores. We have reported that those with a history of suicide attempts score much higher on the Scale for Suicide Ideation than those without such a history (Mann et al. 1999). Furthermore, using a computerized algorithm to devise a recursive decision tree, we have found that subjects with a score of 16 or higher were significantly more likely to have made an attempt at some time in their lives (Mann et al., in press).

Suicide Intent Scale

The Suicide Intent Scale was developed by Beck, Schuyler, and Herman in 1974 (Beck et al. 1974a). This 20-item scale, in which each item is scored between 0 and 2 for severity, has demonstrated good construct validity and reliability (Beck et al. 1974a). It is designed to be administered by a trained clinician during a semistructured interview (Steer et al. 1988). Suicidal intent is measured by assessing the attempter's purpose in making an attempt, how he or she perceived the fatality of the attempt, and how "rescuable" the attempter thought he or she would be (Malone 1996). The Suicide Intent Scale does not include ratings of effectiveness of the attempt, which is measured on the lethality scale and independently of intent.

This scale assesses attempters only (Eyman and Eyman 1992). The first part of the scale covers objective circumstances of the attempt, whereas the second part reflects the attempter's self-report: his or her conceptions of lethality, extent of premeditation, purpose of the attempt, and conceptions of the possibility of rescue. There are four distinct factors that should be measured when assessing suicidal intent. They are 1) attitude toward the attempt (e.g., the attempter's expectations of fatality or lethality and attitude toward dying); 2) planning (e.g., final acts in preparation of death, suicide note); 3) precautions against intervention (e.g., timing, location of attempt, method of attempt); and 4) communication with others (e.g., contacting someone for help).

We have found a positive correlation between planning or suicide intent and medical damage ($r=0.35$; $P<0.005$). This suggests that suicide attempts that result in extensive medical damage are partly the result of careful planning and avoidance of help or medical intervention. A high-planning, high-damage group is likely to be similar to the so-called failed suicide group, or patients who almost completed suicide but survived through good fortune. Similarly, Beck et al. (1975a) found that for patients who accurately assessed the dangerousness of their actions, actual lethality of the suicide attempt increased with intent scores. Of interest, we have also found that intent for the most lethal previous attempt was positively correlated with suicidal ideation immediately before hospital admission ($r=0.624$; $F=9.52$; $df=143,1$;

P=0.002). The intent scale has been correlated with hopelessness and depression (Wetzel et al. 1980), more strongly with hopelessness than with depression (Beck et al. 1974a). These correlations between intent and other parameters that are considered risk factors for suicidal acts are likely to contribute to the robustness of the scale. In fact, higher scores on the Suicide Intent Scale just before suicide completion have been reported as well (Lester et al. 1978), and Beck (1975a) has reported that the mean score on the scale for fatal attempters is higher than for nonfatal attempters.

Medical Lethality

The degree of an individual's intent to kill himself or herself is separate from the medical consequences of the act. Beck et al. (1975a) developed the lethality scale for assessing the degree of medical lethality or damage in a suicide attempt. Intent and lethality are not as highly correlated as one might expect, because attempters often do not accurately assess the lethality of their method. However, the correlation increases when the attempter's preconceptions of the lethality are controlled for in statistical analyses (Beck et al. 1975a). Lethality is rated for eight different methods (e.g., overdose with sedating drugs, cutting, hanging) and on a scale from 0 to 8. A score of 0 signifies that the attempt resulted in no medical damage. For instance, a patient may report taking a small overdose in an effort to kill himself or herself but may suffer no consequences. As the score increases, the medical consequences are more severe, and a score of 8 means that the attempt resulted in death. To our knowledge, the only studies regarding lethality relate to suicide intent (see above).

Hopelessness Scale

The Hopelessness Scale was developed by Beck et al. in 1974 (Beck et al. 1974b). It has 20 true-or-false questions that measure an individual's pessimism about his or her future. Every question that is answered "true" for pessimism is given a score of 1. The total score corresponds to the sum of the individual's pessimistic responses. The scale was designed to obtain three factors: feelings about the future, loss of motivation, and future expectations. The Hopelessness Scale may be useful in assessing and indicating the risk for suicidal behavior in adults (Eyman and Eyman 1992). In one study, a score of 9 or above on the scale was successful in predicting 91% of suicides completed over the subsequent 5–10 years (Beck et al. 1974b). Members of the high-risk group identified by the scale were 11 times more likely to commit suicide than the other patients. Hopelessness is reported to be the best clinical gauge of suicide risk besides a previous suicide attempt (Malone 1996) and is a better indicator of risk than severity of depression as measured by depression scales (Beck et al. 1985; Fawcett et al. 1987). Fawcett et al. (1987) and Drake and Cotton (1986) found that clinical ratings of hopelessness predicted suicide in patients with affective disorders and in those with schizophrenia. The scale has also been found to discriminate among those who communicate suicidal ideation but do not act on it, suicide attempters, and control subjects who do not attempt suicide (Rothberg and Geer-Williams 1992). Furthermore, consistent hopelessness, which remains during treatment, is associated with future suicidal behavior. Together, these studies suggest that high levels of hopelessness are predictors of lifetime suicide risk.

Reasons for Living Inventory

The Reasons for Living (RFL) Inventory (Linehan et al. 1983) evaluates protective factors against suicidal behavior. It is a self-report scale consisting of 48 items. Answers are provided on a scale with six levels, ranging from "not at all important" to "extremely important." The respondent assesses each item (or reason) in terms of degree of importance for killing oneself if suicide were contemplated. These 48 items make up six subscales: Survival and Coping Beliefs (I believe I can learn to adjust or cope with my problems; I have a desire to live), Responsibility to Family (my family might believe I do not love them; I have a responsibility and commitment to my family), Child-Related Concerns (I want to watch my children as they grow; it would not be fair to leave the children for others to take care of), Fear of Suicide (I do not want to die; I am afraid of the unknown), Fear of Social Disapproval (I am concerned about what others would think of me; I would not want people to think I did not have control over my life), and Moral Objections (I believe only God has the right to end a life; my religious beliefs forbid it) (Linehan et al. 1983). Linehan et al. (1983) found that the RFL Inventory differentiated between suicidal and nonsuicidal individuals. The Survival and Coping Beliefs, Responsibility to Family, and Child-Related Concerns factors were the most useful in differentiating between these people. In a study of psychiatric inpatients diagnosed with major depressive disorder, Malone et al. (2000) found that total scores on the RFL Inventory differentiated significantly between suicide attempters and nonattempters. Among the attempters, those with higher scores on items related to moral objections to suicide had lower lethality attempts. We concluded that religious, cultural, and societal factors as assessed in the RFL Inventory functioned as deterrents against acting on suicidal thoughts. This underscores the clinical value of examining protective factors such as reasons for living when assessing suicidal patients.

Conclusions

Assessment of suicide risk cannot be based on results from one scale but instead should take into account risk factors, diagnosis, treatment history, and family history of suicidal behavior. Because typical clinical assessments do not record an individual's suicidal intent and lethality, the clinician commonly overlooks these factors. However, use of scales such as the Columbia Suicide History Form, the Suicide Intent Scale, the Scale for Suicide Ideation, the lethality scale, and the Hopelessness Scale may be one remedy. The use of these semistructured rating scales improves detection of suicidal behavior and risk for suicide. Improved documentation of patients' suicidal behavior, suicidal ideation, suicide intent, and hopelessness will ultimately improve treatment of the suicidal population.

Several caveats exist when assessing an individual's risk for suicide. The ratings scales are reasonable indicators of increased risk for suicidal behavior; however, they are far from foolproof predictors of suicidal acts and give no information about the imminence of the risk. Future research may identify more accurate predictors for suicidal acts and provide clinicians with better tools to assess this life-threatening complication of psychiatric illness.

References

American Psychiatric Association: Diagnostic and Statistical Manual of Mental Disorders, 4th Edition, Text Revision. Washington, DC, American Psychiatric Association, 2000

Asberg M, Traskman L: Studies of CSF 5-HIAA in depression and suicidal behaviour. Adv Exp Med Biol 133:739–752, 1981

Beck AT, Davis JH, Frederick CJ, et al: Classification and nomenclature, in Suicide Prevention in the Seventies. Edited by Resnick HLP, Hathorne BC. Washington, DC, Government Printing Office, 1973, pp 7–12

Beck A, Schuyler D, Herman J: Development of suicidal intent scales, in The Prediction of Suicide. Edited by Beck A, Resnick K, Letierri D. Bowie, MD, Charles Press, 1974a, pp 45–56

Beck AT, Weissman A, Lester D, et al: The measurement of pessimism: the hopelessness scale. J Consult Clin Psychol 42:861–865, 1974b

Beck AT, Beck R, Kovacs M: Classification of suicidal behaviors, I: Quantifying intent and medical lethality. Am J Psychiatry 132:285–287, 1975a

Beck AT, Kovacs M, Weissman A: Hopelessness and suicidal behavior. An overview. JAMA 234:1146–1149, 1975b

Beck AT, Kovacs M, Weissman A: Assessment of suicidal intention: the Scale for Suicide Ideation. J Consult Clin Psychol 47:343–352, 1979

Beck AT, Steer RA, Kovacs M, et al: Hopelessness and eventual suicide: a 10-year prospective study of patients hospitalized with suicidal ideation. Am J Psychiatry 142:559–563, 1985

Beck AT, Steer RA, Ranieri WF: Scale for Suicide Ideation: psychometric properties of a self-report version. J Clin Psychol 44:499–505, 1988

Beck AT, Brown G, Berchick RJ, et al: Relationship between hopelessness and ultimate suicide: a replication with psychiatric outpatients. Am J Psychiatry 147:190–195, 1990

Beck AT, Brown GK, Steer RA, et al: Suicide ideation at its worst point: a predictor of eventual suicide in psychiatric outpatients. Suicide Life Threat Behav 29:1–9, 1999

Brent DA, Oquendo MA, Birmaher B, et al: Familial pathways to early-onset suicide attempt: risk for suicidal behavior in offspring of mood-disordered suicide attempters. Arch Gen Psychiatry 59:801–807, 2002

Brodsky BS, Oquendo MA, Ellis SP, et al: The relationship of childhood abuse to impulsivity and suicidal behavior in adults with major depression. Am J Psychiatry 158:1871–1877, 2001

Chiles JA, Strosahl KD: Assessing suicidal potential. Myths and realities, in The Suicidal Patient. Principles of Assessment, Treatment, and Case Management. Washington, DC, American Psychiatric Press, 1995, pp 35–54

Drake RE, Cotton PG: Depression, hopelessness and suicide in chronic schizophrenia. Br J Psychiatry 148:554–559, 1986

Eyman JR, Eyman SK: Psychological testing for potentially suicidal individuals, in Suicide: Guidelines for Assessment, Management and Treatment. Edited by Bongar B. New York, Oxford University Press, 1992, pp 127–143

Fawcett J, Scheftner W, Clark D, et al: Clinical predictors of suicide in patients with major affective disorders: a controlled prospective study. Am J Psychiatry 144:35–40, 1987

Goldsmith SK, Pellmar TC, Kleinman AM, et al (eds): Reducing Suicide: A National Imperative. Washington, DC, National Academy Press, 2002

Isacsson G, Boethius G, Bergman U: Low level of antidepressant prescription for people who later commit suicide: 15 years of experience from a population-based drug database in Sweden. Acta Psychiatr Scand 85:444–448, 1992

Isometsa ET, Henriksson MM, Aro HM, et al: Suicide in major depression. Am J Psychiatry 151:530–536, 1994

Kamali M, Oquendo MA, Mann JJ: Understanding the neurobiology of suicidal behavior. Depress Anxiety 14:164–176, 2001

Lester D, Beck AT, Narrett S: Suicidal intent in successive suicidal actions. Psychol Rep 43:110, 1978

Linehan MM, Goodstein JL, Nielsen SL, et al: Reasons for staying alive when you are thinking of killing yourself: the reasons for living inventory. J Consult Clin Psychol 51:276–286, 1983

Linnoila M, Virkkunen M, Scheinin M, et al: Low cerebrospinal fluid 5-hydroxyindoleacetic acid concentration differentiates impulsive from non-impulsive violent behavior. Life Sci 33:2609–2614, 1983

Malone KM: Assessment and treatment of suicidal behavior during major depression. Perspectives in Depression 4(3), 1996

Malone KM, Szanto K, Corbitt EM, et al: Clinical assessment versus research methods in the assessment of suicidal behavior. Am J Psychiatry 152:1601–1607, 1995

Malone KM, Oquendo MA, Haas GL, et al: Protective factors against suicidal acts in major depression: reasons for living. Am J Psychiatry 157:1084–1088, 2000

Mann JJ, Malone KM: Cerebrospinal fluid amines and higher lethality suicide attempts in depressed inpatients. Biol Psychiatry 41:162–171, 1997

Mann JJ, Waternaux C, Haas GL, et al: Towards a clinical model of suicidal behavior in psychiatric patients. Am J Psychiatry 156:181–189, 1999

Mann JJ, Liu X, Oquendo MA, et al: Distinguishing past suicide attempters using a classification and regression tree to model clinical decision-making. Am J Psychiatry (in press)

Maris RW, Berman AL, Maltsberger JT, et al (eds): Assessment and Prediction of Suicide. New York, Guilford Press, 1992

Marzuk PM, Tardiff K, Leon AC, et al: The prevalence of aborted suicide attempts among psychiatric in-patients. Acta Psychiatr Scand 96: 492–496, 1997

Miller MC, Jacobs DG, Gutheil TG: Talisman or taboo: the controversy of the suicide-prevention contract. Harv Rev Psychiatry 6:78–87, 1998

National Center for Injury Prevention and Control: Suicide Prevention Fact Sheet. Atlanta, GA, Centers for Disease Control and Prevention, 2002. Available at: http://www.cdc.gov/ncipc/factsheets/suifacts. htm. Accessed December 31, 2002

National Institute of Mental Health: Abstracts of currently funded research grants pertaining to suicidal behavior. Bethesda, MD, National Institute of Mental Health, 2002. Available at: http://www.nimh. nih.gov/research/suiabs.cfm. Accessed December 31, 2002

Nordstrom P, Samuelsson M, Asberg M, et al: CSF 5-HIAA predicts suicide risk after attempted suicide. Suicide Life Threat Behav 24:1–9, 1994

O'Carroll PW, Berman AL, Maris RW, et al: Beyond the Tower of Babel: a nomenclature for suicidology. Suicide Life Threat Behav 26:237–252, 1996

Oquendo MA, Mann JJ: Suicide, in The Encyclopedia of Stress. Edited by Fink G. San Diego, CA, Academic Press, 1999

Oquendo MA, Mann JJ: Un modelo para comprender el riesgo de la conducta suicida: factores neurobiologicos y psicologicos. Psiquiatria 12:40–43, 2000

Oquendo MA, Malone KM, Ellis SP, et al: Inadequacy of antidepressant treatment of patients with major depression who are at risk for suicidal behavior. Am J Psychiatry 156:190–194, 1999

Oquendo MA, Kamali M, Ellis SP, et al: Adequacy of antidepressant treatment after discharge and the occurrence of suicidal acts in major depression: a prospective study. Am J Psychiatry 159:1746–1751, 2002

Pallis DJ, Gibbons JS, Pierce DW: Estimating suicide risk among attempted suicides II. Efficiency of predictive scales after the attempt. Br J Psychiatry 144:139–148, 1984

Pokorny AD: Suicide prediction revisited. Suicide Life Threat Behav 23:1–10, 1993

Rothberg JM, Geer-Williams C: A comparison and review of suicide prediction scales, in Assessment and Prediction of Suicide. Edited by Maris RW, Berman AL, Maltsberger JT, et al. London, Guilford Press, 1992, pp 202–217

Roy A: Risk factors for suicide in psychiatric patients. Arch Gen Psychiatry 39:1089–1095, 1982

Roy A, Segal NL, Sarchiapone M: Attempted suicide among living co-twins of twin suicide victims. Am J Psychiatry 152:1075–1076, 1995

Schulsinger F, Knop J: Social psychiatric research. Heredity, environment, and prevention. Ugeskr Laeger 139:2827–2829, 1977

Stanford EJ, Goetz RR, Bloom JD: The No Harm Contract in the emergency assessment of suicidal risk. J Clin Psychiatry 55:344–348, 1994

Stanley B, Molcho A, Stanley M, et al: Association of aggressive behavior with altered serotonergic function in patients who are not suicidal. Am J Psychiatry 157:609–614, 2000

Statham DJ, Heath AC, Madden PAF, et al: Suicidal behaviour: an epidemiological and genetic study. Psychol Med 28:839–855, 1998

Steer RA, Beck AT, Lester D: Eventual suicide in interrupted and uninterrupted attempters: a challenge to the cry-for-help hypothesis. Suicide Life Threat Behav 18:119–128, 1988

Traskman L, Asberg M, Bertilsson L, et al: Monoamine metabolites in CSF and suicidal behavior. Arch Gen Psychiatry 38:631–636, 1981

Virkkunen M, Rawlings R, Tokola R, et al: CSF biochemistries, glucose metabolism, and diurnal activity rhythms in alcoholic, violent offenders, fire setters, and healthy volunteers. Arch Gen Psychiatry 51:20–27, 1994

Wetzel RD, Margulies T, Davis R, et al: Hopelessness, depression, and suicide intent. J Clin Psychiatry 41:159–160, 1980

SUICIDE HISTORY SUMMARY SCORE SHEET
(To be used with suicide history form)

1. Total number of lifetime actual suicide attempts   _____
2. Total number of ambiguous attempts   _____
3. Total number of interrupted attempts   _____
4. Total number of aborted attempts   _____
5. Highest lethality rating   _____
6. Most recent attempt lethality rating   _____
7. Dates: _____
    First suicide attempt: _____
    Most recent attempt: _____
    Most lethal attempt: _____
8. Lethality of most recent ambiguous attempt   _____ : _____
    (−8=not applicable)
9. Lethality of most lethal ambiguous attempt   _____ : _____
    (−8=not applicable)

SUICIDE HISTORY
Definitions

Actual suicide attempt: A self-injurious act committed with at least some intent to die. Intent does not have to be 100%. If there is any intent to die associated with the act, then it can be considered an actual suicide attempt. Sometimes, even if an individual denies intent, we can infer it clinically from the behavior or circumstances. For example, if someone denies intent to die, but they thought that what they did could be lethal, we often infer intent.

Interrupted attempt: Our definition of an interrupted attempt is when the person is interrupted (by an outside circumstance) from starting the self-injurious act. Here are some examples according to method:
- Overdose: Person has pills in hand but is stopped from ingesting. Once they ingest even one pill, this becomes an attempt rather than an interrupted attempt.
- Shooting: Person has gun pointed toward themselves, gun is taken away by someone else, or is somehow prevented from pulling trigger.
- Jumping: Person is poised to jump, is grabbed and taken down from ledge.
- Hanging: Person has noose around neck but has not yet started to hang—is stopped from doing so.

Aborted attempt: When the person begins to take steps toward making a suicide attempt, but stops themselves before they actually have engaged in any self-destructive behavior. Examples are similar to interrupted attempts, except that the individual stops him/herself, instead of being stopped by someone or something else.

Ambiguous attempt: Refers to a self-injurious attack that looks as if it were done with intent to die, but individual insists that there was no intent to die. In some cases, we can infer intent from the behavior or circumstances, but this definition is reserved for those times when we cannot infer intent. This does not mean that the intent is ambiguous—when intent is ambiguous, we still call it a suicide attempt. We should use this category rarely, if at all.

A SUBJECT IS CONSIDERED AN ATTEMPTER ONLY WHEN WE HAVE DETERMINED THAT THEY HAVE MADE AT LEAST ONE ACTUAL SUICIDE ATTEMPT, AS PER THE ABOVE DEFINITIONS. SOMEONE WHO HAS MADE ONLY AMBIGUOUS, INTERRUPTED, OR ABORTED ATTEMPTS IS NOT CONSIDERED A SUICIDE ATTEMPTER IN OUR STUDY.

CALCULATING IMPRECISION
The IMPRECISION variable indicates how accurate the date of the suicide attempt is, when we do not know the actual date. The number indicates the number of days in the given time period. Interviewers should work with the subject to narrow the date down to the smallest time period possible (week, month, season, year).

- If the subject knows the exact date of the attempt, then IMPRECISION=0
- If the subject can narrow it down to a week, then the date of the attempt is the midpoint of that week, and IMPRECISION=7.
- When you can determine the month, then the date of the attempt is the midpoint of the month (the 15th) and IMPRECISION=30.
- If the subject can tell you the season, here are the midpoint dates for each season:
    > Winter: 2/5
    > Spring: 5/5
    > Summer: 8/5
    > Fall: 11/7

  And IMPRECISION=90.
- The midpoint of any given year is 7/1, and IMPRECISION=365.

HISTORY OF SUICIDAL IDEATION
Have you ever thought of committing suicide?   ___Yes ___ No

How often?   ___ Rarely ___ Sometimes ___ Often   ___ Almost always

When was the last time?_____ DATE: __/__/__

HISTORY/CHRONOLOGY OF SUICIDE ATTEMPTS

1. (IF NOT KNOWN) Did _____ ever attempt suicide?
   [DETERMINE whether there is evidence of any form of   1   2
   self-injurious act with the intent to commit suicide.]   YES   NO
   (INTERVIEWER: if no evidence of possible suicide attempt, STOP, GO TO
   Scale for Suicide Ideation [SSI]. IF YES, CONTINUE.)

2. Total number of lifetime suicide attempts (only self-injurious behavior with intent to die) _____
3. When was the first time he/she ever made an attempt? Please tell me about each, beginning with the first attempt. (TO QUALIFY AS AN ATTEMPT, it is essential to ascertain that there was an intent to die. IF UNCERTAIN, RECORD RELEVANT INFORMATION.)

FOR EACH EVENT ASK: "Tell me exactly what he/she did. What, if any, medical treatments did he/she receive? The aim here is to assess the method used, to obtain an estimate of lethality, and to identify the first, the most lethal, as well as the most recent attempt. [If more than six events, be sure to describe   (1) FIRST ATTEMPT, (2) MOST LETHAL ATTEMPT, and (3) MOST RECENT ATTEMPT.]

BEGIN WITH THE FIRST ATTEMPT:

ATTEMPT # ___ DATE: __ / __ / __ Date Accuracy (± days): ____ **LETHALITY** ____

METHOD code(s): _, _, _ (Number/letter code, see Method code in Leth. Rating Scale; e.g., 1h, 2c, 3e)

ATTEMPT TYPE: 1=Actual 2=Ambiguous 3=Interrupted 4=Aborted

   (a) Please describe for me exactly what happened.

   _____

   (b) If overdose, include names and amount of all substances or drugs:

   _____

   (c) Was he/she alone at the time?   **1=YES**   **2=NO**

   (d) What led up to this event? _____

   _____

If any specific external events appeared to "trigger" the attempt, describe the events and categorize the type of events:

_____

_____

EXTERNAL TRIGGER CATEGORY: ____ (1 to 9 scale) (St. Paul-Ramsey Life Experience Scale) to determine which category the most significant event falls into (1=conjugal, 2=other interpersonal, 3=occupational, 4=living situation, 5=health, 6=other, 7=cannot be assessed, 8=sexual abuse, 9=physical abuse) SECONDARY TRIGGER (category): _____

   (e) What do you think he/she was feeling at the time? _____

   _____

   _____

   (f) Describe any medical consequences of the event (i.e., type of medical damage, including drowsiness, state of consciousness, medical treatment, and response to treatment, and duration of acute condition).

   _____

   _____

Appendix 4–1. Conte Center for the Neuroscience of Mental Disorders/New York State Psychiatric Institute/at Columbia University/Suicide History *(continued)*

ATTEMPT # ___ DATE: __ / __ / __ Date Accuracy (± days): ____ **LETHALITY** ____

METHOD code(s): _, _, _ (Number/letter code, see Method code in Leth. Rating Scale; e.g., 1h, 2c, 3e)

ATTEMPT TYPE: 1=Actual 2=Ambiguous 3=Interrupted 4=Aborted

   (a) Please describe for me exactly what happened.

   (b) If overdose, include names and amount of all substances or drugs:

   (c) Was he/she alone at the time?   **1=YES**   **2=NO**

   (d) What led up to this event? _____

If any specific external events appeared to "trigger" the attempt, describe the events and categorize the type of events:

EXTERNAL TRIGGER CATEGORY: ____ (1 to 9 scale) (St. Paul-Ramsey Life Experience Scale) to determine which category the most significant event falls into (1=conjugal, 2=other interpersonal, 3=occupational, 4=living situation, 5=health, 6=other, 7=cannot be assessed, 8=sexual abuse, 9=physical abuse)

SECONDARY TRIGGER (category): _____

   (e) What do you think he/she was feeling at the time? _____

   (f) Describe any medical consequences of the event (i.e., type of medical damage, including drowsiness, state of consciousness, medical treatment, and response to treatment, and duration of acute condition).

ATTEMPT # ___ DATE: __ / __ / __ Date Accuracy (± days): ____ **LETHALITY** ____

METHOD code(s): _, _, _ (Number/letter code, see Method code in Leth. Rating Scale; e.g., 1h, 2c, 3e)

ATTEMPT TYPE: 1=Actual 2=Ambiguous 3=Interrupted 4=Aborted

   (a) Please describe for me exactly what happened.

   (b) If overdose, include names and amount of all substances or drugs:

   (c) Was he/she alone at the time?   **1=YES**   **2=NO**

   (d) What led up to this event? _____

Appendix 4–1. Conte Center for the Neuroscience of Mental Disorders/New York State Psychiatric Institute/at Columbia University/Suicide History *(continued)*

If any specific external events appeared to "trigger" the attempt, describe the events and categorize the type of events:

_____

_____

EXTERNAL TRIGGER CATEGORY: _____ (1 to 9 scale) (St. Paul-Ramsey Life Experience Scale) to determine which category the most significant event falls into (1=conjugal, 2=other interpersonal, 3=occupational, 4=living situation, 5=health, 6=other, 7=cannot be assessed, 8=sexual abuse, 9=physical abuse) SECONDARY TRIGGER (category): _____

   (e) What do you think he/she was feeling at the time? _____

     _____

     _____

   (f) Describe any medical consequences of the event (i.e., type of medical damage, including drowsiness, state of consciousness, medical treatment, and response to treatment, and duration of acute condition).

     _____

     _____

ATTEMPT # ___ DATE: __ /__ /__ Date Accuracy (± days): ____ **LETHALITY** ____

METHOD code(s): _, _, _ (Number/letter code, see Method code in Leth. Rating Scale; e.g., 1h, 2c, 3e)

ATTEMPT TYPE: 1=Actual 2=Ambiguous 3=Interrupted 4=Aborted

   (a) Please describe for me exactly what happened.

     _____

   (b) If overdose, include names and amount of all substances or drugs:

     _____

   (c) Was he/she alone at the time?   **1=YES**   **2=NO**

   (d) What led up to this event? _____

     _____

If any specific external events appeared to "trigger" the attempt, describe the events and categorize the type of events:

_____

_____

EXTERNAL TRIGGER CATEGORY: _____ (1 to 9 scale) (St. Paul-Ramsey Life Experience Scale) to determine which category the most significant event falls into (1=conjugal, 2=other interpersonal, 3=occupational, 4=living situation, 5=health, 6=other, 7=cannot be assessed, 8=sexual abuse, 9=physical abuse) SECONDARY TRIGGER (category): _____

   (e) What do you think he/she was feeling at the time? _____

     _____

     _____

(f) Describe any medical consequences of the event (i.e., type of medical damage, including drowsiness, state of consciousness, medical treatment, and response to treatment, and duration of acute condition).

ATTEMPT # ___ DATE: __ / __ / __ Date Accuracy (± days): ____ **LETHALITY** ____

METHOD code(s): _, _, _ (Number/letter code, see Method code in Leth. Rating Scale; e.g., 1h, 2c, 3e)

ATTEMPT TYPE: 1=Actual 2=Ambiguous 3=Interrupted 4=Aborted

(a) Please describe for me exactly what happened.

(b) If overdose, include names and amount of all substances or drugs:

(c) Was he/she alone at the time?   1=YES   2=NO

(d) What led up to this event? _____

If any specific external events appeared to "trigger" the attempt, describe the events and categorize the type of events:

EXTERNAL TRIGGER CATEGORY: ____ (1 to 9 scale) (St. Paul-Ramsey Life Experience Scale) to determine which category the most significant event falls into (1=conjugal, 2=other interpersonal, 3=occupational, 4=living situation, 5=health, 6=other, 7=cannot be assessed, 8=sexual abuse, 9=physical abuse)

SECONDARY TRIGGER (category): _____

(e) What do you think he/she was feeling at the time? _____

(f) Describe any medical consequences of the event (i.e., type of medical damage, including drowsiness, state of consciousness, medical treatment, and response to treatment, and duration of acute condition).

ATTEMPT # ___ DATE: __ / __ / __ Date Accuracy (± days): ____ **LETHALITY** ____

METHOD code(s): _, _, _ (Number/letter code, see Method code in Leth. Rating Scale; e.g., 1h, 2c, 3e)

ATTEMPT TYPE: 1=Actual 2=Ambiguous 3=Interrupted 4=Aborted

(a) Please describe for me exactly what happened.

   (b) If overdose, include names and amount of all substances or drugs:

   (c) Was he/she alone at the time?   **1=YES**   **2=NO**

   (d) What led up to this event? _____

If any specific external events appeared to "trigger" the attempt, describe the events and categorize the type of events:

EXTERNAL TRIGGER CATEGORY: ____ (1 to 9 scale) (St. Paul-Ramsey Life Experience Scale) to determine which category the most significant event falls into (1=conjugal, 2=other interpersonal, 3=occupational, 4=living situation, 5=health, 6=other, 7=cannot be assessed, 8=sexual abuse, 9=physical abuse) SECONDARY TRIGGER (category): _____

   (e) What do you think he/she was feeling at the time? _____

   (f) Describe any medical consequences of the event (i.e., type of medical damage, including drowsiness, state of consciousness, medical treatment, and response to treatment, and duration of acute condition).

NOTE: ADD EXTRA SUICIDE HISTORY PAGES TO INCLUDE ALL SUICIDE ATTEMPTS.

Chapter 5

Nationwide Implementation of Global Assessment of Functioning as an Indicator of Patient Severity and Service Outcomes

William W. Van Stone, M.D.
Kathy L. Henderson, M.D.
Rudolf H. Moos, Ph.D.
Robert Rosenheck, M.D.
Mary Schohn, Ph.D.

The Global Assessment of Functioning (GAF) scale is a standard part (i.e., Axis V) of the American Psychiatric Association's multiaxial system included in DSM-IV-TR (American Psychiatric Association 2000) and has been used optionally since 1977 as part of the recording of a mental health diagnosis in U.S. Department of Veterans Affairs (VA) clinical settings.

Since 1997, VA policy has required clinicians to use the GAF as part of the diagnostic system for all mental health inpatients and outpatients. Two developments led to this policy. First, in 1995, the Government Performance Results Act of 1993 (P.L. 103-62) mandated all federal agencies to measure functional outcomes. The law permitted the VA to use the GAF at a national level to determine whether VA mental health services produced demonstrable improvements in patients' functioning and symptoms.

Second, the Veterans Healthcare Eligibility Reform Act of 1996 (P.L. 104-262) required the Veterans Health Administration (VHA) to "maintain its capacity to provide for the specialized treatment and rehabilitation needs of disabled veterans (including those with...mental illness)." VA decided to use the GAF to define which patients with a mental illness were officially disabled, in line with a definition from the *Federal Register* (Federal Register 1993, p. 29425) that a "disability is a functional impairment that substantially interferes with or limits one or more major life activities, including basic daily living skills, instrumental living skills, and/or vocational and education activities." A national consensus independent of the VA suggested that a GAF score of 50 or under defined serious mental illness (National Advisory Mental Health Council 1993).

The GAF seemed to be an ideal procedure to measure treatment outcomes and to serve as a severity indicator for serious mental illness for the capacity report. It required little time from busy clinicians who were already familiar with their patients, training was thought to be unnecessary because the GAF had been part of DSM-III-R and DSM-IV (American Psychiatric Association 1987, 1994) multiaxial evaluation since 1987, and the GAF was designed to measure both levels of functioning and symptoms. Accordingly, in November 1997, a VA policy directive stated that "as part of the diagnosis, mental health clinicians are required to record at least one GAF score...for each veteran patient seen at any VHA mental health inpatient or outpatient setting" (U.S. Department of Veterans Affairs 1997, p. 2).

Implementing Use of the GAF Throughout the Veterans Health Administration

For several decades, the VA has used computerized patient records systems in each facility. A mental health package has been part of this system since the beginning. In addition, there is a central database in Austin, Texas, that stores items selected from each facility computer system, which are used to analyze workload or cost data at the regional network or national level. To make a proposal such as obtaining a GAF rating on all mental health patients feasible in this large decentralized system, the VA needed, at a minimum, the following elements (Figure 5–1):

- The cooperation of the clinicians who provide and record GAF ratings on their patients.
- An electronic record that would include the GAF rating, the name of the clinician doing the rating, and the date of the rating (the event).
- An electronic storage file at each facility to store each event.
- A method to systematically transfer summary information to the nationwide VA database and check it for accuracy.
- Software that could extract data from the nationwide data files, combine it with other related information, and produce and distribute the summary information.
- The ongoing cooperation of the administrative and information system staff at each facility so that the system would be maintained and national data would be complete and accurate.

GAF as an Outcome Measure

Once the software was developed and tested, the VA initiated a national performance measure (an incentive system tied in with the 21 network directors' bonuses and ratings) to ensure that the GAF was performed on all mental health patients and that the results were recorded and transmitted to the central database. With the use of monitors published monthly, the number of patients eligible for the GAF who had a GAF score recorded in the national database gradually increased from an average for all networks of 46% in 1998 (range, 15%–65%) to 66% in fiscal year (FY) 2002 (range, 33%–90%). Accordingly, when incentive systems are in place, high rates of compliance in using the GAF can be obtained.

Lessons Learned

The VA learned a number of lessons during the implementation effort. First, it typically takes much longer than expected to develop, test, and field new software, especially at the national

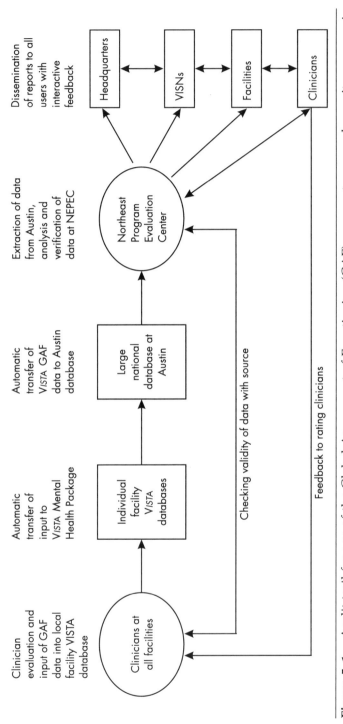

Figure 5–1. Audit trail for use of the Global Assessment of Functioning (GAF) as an outcome and severity measure in Veterans Health Administration (VHA) facilities.

Note. VISTA (formerly DHCP) is the name of the main computer program at each VHA facility; NEPEC=Northeast Program Evaluation Center (at West Haven VA Medical Center); VISNs=Veterans Integrated Services Networks.

multisite level. In addition, monitoring must be ongoing, and it is expensive. Second, in a complex health care system, the will and ability to comply with a new clinical monitoring system vary at each facility. Ongoing monitoring and monthly feedback—especially in the context of specific performance incentives—can be effective. Third, if a proposal for a clinical measure has a plausible rationale, is not time consuming, and is supported by management, clinicians tend to comply.

Staff Involvement and Training in One VA Network

In FY 1997, the Upstate New York VA Network (one of 21 throughout the nation) began developing a care line structure for the delivery of all health care services. In behavioral health, this meant a move toward a structure in which all behavioral health providers and support staff operated under one regionally based management team. The change in organizational structure was accompanied by a change in organizational philosophy. The new organizational vision was based not just on improving the quality of health care for veterans but also on providing empirical evidence of these improvements. At a national level, VA headquarters was beginning to define and prescribe specific outcome measures for this purpose. The GAF was one of the first measures proposed for use in evaluating behavioral health programs.

Development of GAF Training

In the fall of FY 1997, Dr. Scott Murray, director of the Behavioral Health Care Line, identified a clinical champion to develop and oversee a clinical task force on the GAF. The charge to the task force was to review the literature on the GAF, identify or develop training materials, identify and implement a training process that was inexpensive but accessible to clinicians at all five sites, and develop a process to meet the performance standard established by the VHA.

The task group decided that a standardized approach to training was required, with additional explicit instructions in scoring. Instructions for scoring the GAF in the 1997 user's guide for the Structured Clinical Interview for DSM-IV Axis I Disorders (First et al. 1997) were used as the basis for training. The group also identified clinical vignettes for both training and evaluating the success of the training program. Finally, they obtained information about the data entry issues related to capturing the GAF for the database. The resulting training packet consisted of a pretest, a posttest, several clinical vignettes that covered a range of GAF scores, literature on the use of the GAF, scoring instructions, data entry instructions, and the GAF scale itself.

The training was structured to last no more than 90 minutes, with the caveat that ongoing practice was required. After completion of a pretest to provide a baseline to estimate the reliability of the GAF, the rules for scoring were presented and the staff was divided into subgroups to begin scoring the training vignettes. When the subgroups completed the task, the whole group reconvened to discuss issues and concerns that arose in assigning the scores. Through this discussion, staff members soon realized that the GAF was reliable when everyone used the same scoring rules. Finally a posttest was given for later review by training staff.

The initial training improved the reliability of the use of the GAF. The most significant finding was that untrained clinicians tended to assign a GAF score that was too high, apparently because they thought that a low GAF score was a negative reflection on a patient rather than a true measure of functioning. A second finding was that vignettes that contained more information were more reliably scored by clinicians. This suggested that for a single patient there might be variations in GAF score between a single assessment performed by an arbitrary provider and one performed by a more permanent provider.

The task force also identified system issues, such as how to provide ongoing training in a large organization with staff turnover and extensive multidisciplinary training programs, and how to ensure that the data entry component of the process was reliable and easy for clinicians to use.

In the final training program, the task force recommended that the primary outpatient therapist assume responsibility for performing the GAF. If this was not possible, they recommended that every GAF score assignment should occur concurrently with a written progress note that detailed the basis on which the score was assigned. Second, they recommended that each clinical program begin discussion of the assignment of the GAF as a routine part of treatment team reviews. Finally, they recommended a change in the billing form to permit the clinician to enter the GAF score on the form for data entry by clerical staff.

Implementation of the training occurred between December 1998 and February 1999. Through the diligence of 10 trainers, the task force reached more than 400 clinical staff members in the Behavioral Health Care Line. Based on the pretesting and posttesting, the average clinician moved from scoring two of five vignettes correctly to four of five. As the training task group reviewed these gains, they noted that trained staff members tended to improve but sometimes needed additional training. Although the consistency of scores improved, review of the database indicated that problems in reliability still remained, especially between inpatient discharge scores and the first outpatient appointment. Behavioral health clinicians were retested in the summer of 2000 to see how well training gains were maintained. Review of these data suggested that trained staff members continued to assign reliable scores, but new staff members were not being trained adequately. By the end of FY 2000, the Upstate New York Network was one of the leaders in the VA on the GAF performance measure.

Successful Implementation of GAF Scores in the Most Populous VA Network

The South Central VA Health Care Network has been successful in integrating the GAF scale into the everyday practice of mental health providers. The South Central Network is the largest of the 21 Veterans Integrated Services Networks (VISNs) as measured by veteran population (1.8 million) and has the second-largest unique number of veterans treated at its health care facilities (more than 350,000 treated in 2001). In addition, this network (VISN 16) covers a vast area, providing health care to veterans in Oklahoma, Arkansas, Louisiana, Mississippi, and parts of Texas,

Missouri, Alabama, and Florida; it includes 10 medical centers, 30 community-based outpatient clinics, 2 domiciliaries, and 7 nursing homes. The network thus faced a major challenge in implementing the nationally mandated GAF protocol.

In 1997, the VISN established a network-wide Mental Health Product Line (MHPL). This organizational structure was designed to more effectively coordinate the delivery of mental health services throughout the VISN. One of its missions includes monitoring national and network-wide mental health performance measures and assisting facilities in compliance with these measures. Before the formation of a network-level mental health organization, each facility worked independently to implement and monitor these measures. Although there had been a preexisting mental health workgroup in the network, in 1998 the MHPL organized a mental health advisory council, which was composed of the mental health managers from the 10 medical centers. Together, these two structures have set priorities for mental health programs across the network. The working relationship of these two bodies has been instrumental in achieving the success in implementing the GAF as an outcome measure.

Most mental health providers were aware of VHA Directive 97-059 (U.S. Department of Veterans Affairs 1997, p. 2) requiring a recording of "at least one GAF score…for each veteran patient seen at any VHA mental health inpatient or outpatient setting." However, in FY 1998 the National Mental Health Program Monitoring System (Rosenheck and DiLella 1999) measured the performance of VISN 16 as 57% (range per facility, 0%–78%). The impetus to improve performance came in 1999 when a national performance measure was developed stating that mental health patients seen during a 90-day period (one quarter) on either an inpatient or an outpatient basis should have at least one GAF score recorded in that same quarter.

At the time of the introduction of this measure, the network's performance was approximately 60%. It was a tremendous challenge to meet the network's targeted goal of 90%, which was achieved in FY 2002. To achieve the goal, the MHPL enlisted the support of the VISN 16 Information Technology Development Group to develop a user-friendly computer program that would provide the facilities with the data needed to monitor and improve their performance on this measure.

The software, written by a VISN programmer and installed on each facility's local computer system, gives each user the ability to identify which patients have had GAFs completed and which had not. The program produces two reports of the GAF monitor:

- The first report provides the numerator (patients with a GAF), the denominator (number of unique inpatients and outpatients), and the percentage of GAFs to the total number of patients.
- The second report is a listing of patients who have not received a GAF. It provides the patient's name, social security number, date of stay or encounter, and hospital ward or clinic. This report is sorted by individual providers.

The reports are sent via hospital e-mail to recipients in the mental health mail group who can then take proactive measures to obtain GAFs for patients on the outlier list. These reports can be accessed for any date range and can be run as frequently as requested by the provider. In addition, monthly reports by facility using the same program are monitored by the MHPL, and the results are distributed to each facility for comparison and review.

Additional interventions were also employed to improve GAF data collection. For example, education of mental health providers was conducted at both the network and the facility level using clinical vignettes to improve scoring reliability. Policies were instituted at the facility level stating that GAFs will be completed on all mental health patients at each visit and will be documented in the progress note. Some facilities instituted the GAF within the clinical reminder package to prompt providers when GAFs are due. The most important element for success appears to be the personal feedback by the service chief to individual mental health providers when their patients are listed as outliers. As a result of these combined efforts, within 1 year VISN 16 had improved its performance in GAF documentation from 60% to 82%. In subsequent years scores continued to improve, with network averages of 88%–90%. Several of the medical centers consistently score 95%–97% completion rates.

National GAF Training by Satellite Broadcast

The training experience garnered by these two networks was also echoed at the national level. During July and August 2001, on three occasions the VA Employee Education System (EES) broadcast satellite training programs to all VA facilities regarding use of the GAF. EES subsequently made training videotapes available for distribution.

Working with several clinicians experienced in training mental health professionals in performing reliable GAFs as well as with Dr. Michael First, who is a major advocate for the GAF systems, EES devised a national training program using the VA national satellite broadcast system, available at all VA facilities. The program provided a review of the GAF as it applies in the VA and how, when interpreted uniformly, GAF scores can be used as a professional and reliable tool for assessing the level of functioning in mental health patients.

The training emphasized the following issues:

- GAF score reflects the *lowest* level of either symptoms or functioning over a specified period of time. For outpatients it is typically the lowest level during the past week; for inpatients it is the lowest level in the recent past that reflects the need for hospitalization.
- The GAF score always reflects the domain in which the worst symptoms or functioning occurs despite possibly better functioning in other domains.
- A patient's GAF score is within the lowest 10-point range when either the symptom severity or level of functioning falls within that range.
- A four-step method is used for descending down the GAF scale to get at the right score.

In addition, the faculty noted common errors in conceptualizing the GAF as well as in determining the actual scores.

Feedback forms were received from 712 individuals who attended one of the broadcasts in 86 VA facilities. Comments were generally favorable and frequently noted that the clinicians had been rating their patients much too high.

Preliminary Analysis of GAF Outcomes

Although improvements in the use of the GAF as a rating instrument in the VA clearly need to continue, the VA Northeast Program Evaluation Center has conducted preliminary analyses of the available data to demonstrate ways in which GAF data may eventually be used to describe outcomes across the 21 VA networks. In FY 2000, VA clinicians documented well over 500,000 GAF ratings for more than 250,000 veterans. However, follow-up GAF scores were collected on only 164,000 veterans, just 31% of veterans with two or more visits.

Although the available data are therefore incomplete, it is possible to explore ways of using GAF data to measure outcomes across the VA system. Because the goal is to examine outcomes, the central measure is a simple one: the change in GAF score between a baseline time point and a later follow-up time point, calculated simply as the "post" rating minus the "pre" rating.

It might seem natural and desirable to obtain a GAF score at the very beginning of treatment, but identifying a clear beginning is almost impossible in most cases, because so many VA patients have been in and out of the system for long periods of time. Instead, outcomes are measured as they occur, using shifting baselines along the way. There is another reason for *not* identifying a single beginning. As a subjective clinical assessment, the GAF is highly subject to rater bias. In other words it is "fudgeable." If VISNs are being compared, it would be natural to rate the baseline status as low as possible, to leave maximal room for improvement, and the follow-up status as high as possible, so that improvement ratings could be maximized. Such bias in ratings would most likely be unavoidable in the increasingly competitive environment.

The solution proposed to this dilemma is to have shifting baselines, so that a rater does not know if any given rating will be used as a baseline or follow-up rating. The best option, therefore, is to do an accurate rating. Six different change measures have been developed; two involve inpatient care and four involve out-patient care.

1. The first measure uses an inpatient GAF score as the baseline and an outpatient GAF score obtained between 2 and 6 months after discharge as the follow-up (Table 5–1). The average change (i.e., follow-up minus baseline) on this measure was 4.9 in points in FY 2000, with a range across VISNs from 11.0 to 1.6.
2. The second measure again uses an inpatient GAF score as the baseline, but then uses the *last* GAF score of the year for that patient, to show maximal improvement (Table 5–1). The aver-age improvement on this measure was 6.4, with a range across VISNs from 10.1 to 2.8. It should be noted that in this longer follow-up period, there is more improvement. Time heals.

The next three measures are based on changes between out-patient GAF assessments (Table 5–1):

1. The first outpatient measure addresses change from the first GAF score of the year to the last GAF score obtained in the fol-lowing 6 months.
2. The second measure records the change from the first GAF score to the last GAF score of the year.
3. The third measure records the change from the first GAF score in the second half of the year to the last GAF score of the year.

These outpatient GAF scores show little change, with a mean gain of about 0.4 GAF points and a VISN maximum of about 5 and a minimum of −1, reflecting the stable status of most out-patients on average.

1. The final measure is the change in GAF score in newly admit-ted outpatients, defined as those with no outpatient visit at all during the first 3 months of the year. The average improve-ment on this measure was 1.9, just between the 5-point improvement in inpatients and the 0.4 improvement in outpa-tients. The range across VISNs was 4.6 to −0.41.

Table 5–1. Change scores: inpatient to outpatient and outpatient to outpatient

	VISN	
	Mean	**Max. to Min.**
Inpatient to outpatient		
2- to 6-month follow-up	4.9	11.0 to 1.6
Last GAF of the year	6.4	10.1 to 2.8
Outpatient to outpatient		
1st 6-month GAF to last GAF of 6 months	0.46	2.6 to 1.1
1st 6-month GAF to last GAF of year	0.33	4.6 to −1.0
2nd 6-month GAF to last GAF of 6 months	0.38	2.6 to −0.66
1st GAF of episode to last GAF of year	1.9	4.6 to −0.41

Note. GAF=Global Assessment of Functioning; VISN=Veterans Integrated Services Network.

One additional issue must be considered before using these measures to compare outcomes across VISNs. There are differences across VISNs in patient mix—in characteristics such as age, diagnosis, service connection, etc.—and these factors can influence GAF outcomes.

For example, looking at diagnostic groups (Table 5–2), patients with Alzheimer's disease, schizophrenia, and PTSD have poorer outcomes (by about 2 points) than other patients, whereas patients with anxiety disorders, dysthymic disorder, or adjustment disorder have better outcomes (by about a half-point).

Age, in contrast, has little effect on outcomes (Table 5–3). However, minorities show less improvement than whites, as do veterans who received VA compensation for service-related disabilities rated at 50% or more. Veterans with service-connected disabilities less than 50%, in contrast, have better outcomes.

In addition, veterans with high baseline GAF scores show less improvement—most likely because of the phenomenon of regression to the mean: patients who start with high scores are likely to see declines and vice versa. It also turns out that VISNs with better representation of their outpatients in the GAF files have better outcomes. In other words, VISNs in which a larger percentage of patients had at least two mental health outpatient

Table 5–2. Diagnostic predictors of change in Global Assessment of Functioning score (all $P<0.0001$)

	Regression coefficient
Alzheimer's disease	−2.7
Schizophrenia	−2.8
Posttraumatic stress disorder	−2.4
Drug abuse/dependency	−0.91
Alcohol abuse/dependency	−0.74
Bipolar disorder	−0.40
Anxiety disorder	+0.21
Dysthymia	+0.29
Adjustment disorder	+0.56

Table 5–3. Other predictors of change in Global Assessment of Functioning (GAF) score

	Regression coefficient	P
Age	−0.003	NS
Black	−0.18	0.05
Hispanic	−0.59	0.0001
Service-connected disability 100%	−1.42	0.001
Service-connected disability 50%–90%	−0.41	0.0001
Service-connected disability 10%–40%	+0.59	0.0001
Baseline GAF	−0.45	0.0001
Percent with GAF follow-up (per 10%)	+0.45	0.0001

clinic visits had more usable GAF change scores and showed better outcomes.

Statistical models of change can be used to control for all of these differences. This procedure, called risk adjustment, levels the playing field as much as possible in comparing performance across the VISNs.

In the final analysis, there are six risk-adjusted, average GAF change scores for each VISN. These could then be averaged to give a final summary outcome performance score.

It is notable that when scores are averaged at the VISN level, these six measures are highly correlated with one another, with correlation coefficients ranging from 0.62 to 0.97 (Table 5–4). Cronbach's α is a statistic that measures how much a set of measures is getting at the same underlying construct. That these six measures of GAF change have a Cronbach's α of 0.90 (quite high) means that they are measuring a common construct—presumably the amount of clinical improvement in VA mental health patients. Thus, although the six measures are quite different, the differences they show between VA networks are pretty consistent across the different measures. This suggests that they have some degree of reliability and perhaps validity. If the scores were totally arbitrary, one would not expect to find such high correlations.

Conclusions

Two broad sets of conclusions can be drawn from these analyses. First, these analyses suggest that even though training in the use of the GAF across the VA system is incomplete and uneven, when data from large numbers of patients are analyzed many expected patterns are seen. For instance, although there is substantial improvement through the transition from inpatient to outpatient, *on average* outpatients tend to remain stable, although newly admitted outpatients show four times as much improvement as continuing patients. Diagnostic and sociodemographic patterns are also consistent with expectations, although the observation of poorer outcomes among minorities is cause for concern.

Table 5–4. Correlation of VA network GAF change scores

	2	3	4	5	6
4-month follow-up (IP)	0.89	0.53	0.53	0.57	0.58
Last GAF of the year (IP)		0.66	0.63	0.68	0.68
1st 6-month GAF to last 6-month GAF (OP)			0.97	0.88	0.70
1st 6-month GAF to last GAF of year (OP)				0.91	0.67
2nd 6-month GAF to last 6-month GAF (OP)					0.62
1st GAF of episode to last GAF of year (OP)					

Note. Internal consistency (Cronbach's α)=0.90. Abbreviations: IP=inpatient; OP=outpatient.

Second, after risk adjustment, different measures have similar relationships across VISNs. This suggests that when used with large numbers of patients the GAF may eventually be a useful tool for evaluating and comparing global outcomes in the VA and other large health care systems.

The GAF, Mental Health Service Use, and Patients' Symptom and Functioning Outcomes

As part of the VA's nationwide outcomes monitoring program, the GAF data were used to address four questions:

- Are clinicians' GAF ratings relatively reliable?
- Are GAF ratings closely associated with other measures of patients' social and occupational functioning?
- Are GAF ratings closely associated with patients' receipt of mental health services; that is, do more impaired patients receive more care?
- Do GAF ratings predict patients' symptom and social or occupational treatment outcomes?

Two studies were conducted to examine these questions. One study focused on 1,688 patients who were administered the GAF as inpatients and were included in a VA-based evaluation of three distinctive treatments for patients with substance use disorders (Ouimette et al. 1997). These patients were assessed at baseline and 1 year later on three indices of psychological functioning (emotional distress, psychiatric symptoms, and substance use problems), three indices of social functioning (residential stability, number of friends, and quality of relationships with friends), and two indices of occupational functioning (employment status and annual income) (Moos et al. 2000).

The second study took advantage of the fact that the VA mandated the use of the Addiction Severity Index (ASI) (McLellan et al. 1992) in an outcomes monitoring program to assess all patients with a substance use disorder—including those with a comorbid psychiatric disorder—at entry into treatment and at a 6- to 12-month follow-up. In the first phase of this program, clinicians used the GAF to rate 9,854 patients in 148 VA facilities who had also undergone baseline and follow-up evaluation with the ASI (Moos et al. 2002). The ASI items were used to assess three symptom-related outcomes (psychiatric symptoms, alcohol and drug use, and substance use problems) and four social and occupational functioning outcomes (family and social problems, the presence of one or more close friends, legal problems, and employment status).

The second study examined the association between GAF ratings and the services patients received. Information obtained from the VA National Patient Care Database was used to specify an index episode of mental health care for each patient. The information covered specific services in the index episode: whether or not the patient had inpatient or residential care, and if so, the number of days of care; whether or not the patient had outpatient mental health or medical care, and if so, the number of visits for psychiatric, substance abuse, and medical care.

The findings from these studies support the following four conclusions, at least with respect to veteran patients being treated for substance use disorders:

1. Clinicians showed high agreement in their GAF ratings.

   Clinicians completed two separate GAF ratings within seven days on 1,175 patients included in the second study. The agreement between the two ratings was quite high (a correlation of 0.80). Thus, clinicians agreed quite well in their routine GAF ratings of patients' impairment; in fact, the level of agreement was somewhat higher than that shown in some previous studies (Fernando et al. 1986; Howes et al. 1997; Loevdahl and Friis 1996).

2. Clinicians' GAF ratings were somewhat associated with patients' diagnoses and symptom severity, but they were only minimally associated with patients' social and occupational functioning as measured by other indices.

   In DSM-III-R and DSM-IV, ratings of global functioning are included as Axis V to obtain an estimate of impairment that adds to already available information about a patient's diagnosis and symptom severity. However, in both studies, clinicians' ratings of patients' global impairment were more closely associated with patients' diagnoses, prior treatment, and symptom severity than with their social or occupational functioning. Patients with psychiatric diagnoses, psychoses, and recent prior inpatient care were rated as more impaired, as were patients who reported more psychiatric symptoms and substance use problems. Once these clinical and symptom factors were considered, indices of social and occupational functioning added only a negligible amount of predictable variance to GAF ratings.

These findings support earlier work showing moderately robust associations between patients' symptoms and GAF ratings (Coulehan et al. 1997; Hall 1995; Mueser et al. 1997; Van Gastel et al. 1997). They indicate that these ratings contain little if any information about patients' social or occupational functioning that is independent of clinicians' judgments about patients' diagnoses and the severity of their symptoms (Brekke 1992; Roy-Byrne et al. 1996; Skodol et al. 1988).

3. Clinicians' GAF ratings were not closely associated with patients' receipt of services in an index episode of care, as measured by the VA patient care databases.

More-impaired patients were more likely to receive inpatient or residential care; however, less-impaired patients received as much inpatient or residential care as did more-impaired patients. More-impaired patients also were somewhat more likely to receive outpatient psychiatric care, but they did not receive more psychiatric care. Moreover, more-impaired patients were less likely to receive outpatient substance abuse care, and they received somewhat less such care than less-impaired patients did.

Outpatient medical care did not substitute for mental health care: more-impaired patients were no more likely than their less-impaired counterparts to obtain outpatient medical care, and they obtained somewhat less medical care. Overall, patients who were rated as having more serious or pervasive impairment had shorter episodes of care than did patients with less impairment. Thus, with the exception of inpatient and residential and outpatient psychiatric care, global impairment ratings either were not associated with the allocation of services or showed that more-impaired patients received fewer services.

4. Clinicians' GAF ratings were not closely associated with patients' symptom or social and occupational functioning outcomes.

There was little if any relationship between ratings of patients' global functioning and their symptom or social/occupational outcomes. In the first study, only minimal associations were identified between clinicians' ratings of patients' current level of functioning and patients' self-rated symptoms and functioning at treatment outcome. This finding was replicated in the second study and was extended to encompass treatment outcome as based on clinicians' interviews.

Conclusions and Next Steps

The GAF ratings were highly reliable and there was some evidence of their validity, because patients with more severe psychiatric diagnoses, current inpatient or residential care, and more psychiatric symptoms and substance use problems were likely to be rated as being more impaired. However, consistent with earlier studies (Dufton and Siddique 1992; Goldman et al. 1992; Piersma and Boes 1995; C. W. Sullivan and Grubia 1991), the findings cast doubt on the value of GAF ratings as predictors of mental health service use or longer-term treatment outcome. Although it is intuitively appealing, a brief rating of global functioning may not be able to capture changes in psychological, social, and occupational functioning that at best are only moderately interrelated (Dohrenwend et al. 1983; Moos et al. 2000; Strauss and Carpenter 1977).

It is important to recognize that the findings reflect the use of the GAF in a nationwide system of care comprising many different clinicians with varying levels of experience and expertise. The GAF ratings were not obtained under controlled conditions with specific training to enhance validity, such as through the use of a validity check on vignettes of patients with known levels of impairment or the use of experts' ratings of a subset of patients. Further studies are needed to determine whether more extensive training and use of experts' ratings can enhance the value of the GAF as a predictor of treatment allocation and outcome, and whether comparing initial and follow-up GAF scores can index program effectiveness. Comparative studies of the GAF and potential alternative assessment procedures (American Psychiatric Association 1994; Johnston and Pollard 2001; Patterson and Lee 1995; Robert et al. 1991; Stewart and Ware 1992; G. Sullivan et al. 2001) may help to identify clinically valid measures that tap patients' psychosocial functioning in a way that adds some unique information to what is already known about their diagnoses and symptoms.

The GAF is an attractive part of an outcomes monitoring system because it is simple and easy to use, but it may have some conceptual and empirical limitations. Moreover, it is based solely on clinicians' in-treatment assessments, whereas to obtain an adequate assessment of the outcome of care, it is useful to obtain some information directly from patients, especially after they have completed treatment. It is not yet clear whether a more complex assessment procedure can obtain predictive information about the use of mental health services or treatment outcome that adds to the GAF in an efficient and cost-effective manner. The VA's experience with the GAF and other outcomes monitoring procedures should help to answer this question and lead to improved ways of measuring the quality and outcome of mental health services both in the VA and in the broader mental health care community.

The paradox remains that the more accurate and meaningful measures of outcome cost in the many hundreds of dollars for each patient, whereas the inexpensive measures that can be taken from extensive databases may suggest some aspects of the process of treatment (such as hospitalization rates) but are still far away from providing credible information about the effectiveness of treatments for individuals or even groups of patients. Attempts to create outcome measures for patients with a specific diagnosis are also being explored. Systematic chart review using sampling techniques is another approach that has worked well in the general medical field and is being developed for mental healthcare in the VA.

The bottom line is that so far, the GAF is the most cost-effective method available to provide a global indication of how patients are functioning and what the level of their symptoms is over time. It will most likely continue to be one part of a series of measures suggesting the effectiveness of mental health treatment in the VA.

References

American Psychiatric Association: Diagnostic and Statistical Manual of Mental Disorders, 3rd Edition, Revised. Washington, DC, American Psychiatric Association, 1987

American Psychiatric Association: Diagnostic and Statistical Manual of Mental Disorders, 4th Edition. Washington, DC, American Psychiatric Association, 1994

American Psychiatric Association: Diagnostic and Statistical Manual of Mental Disorders, 4th Edition, Text Revision. Washington, DC, American Psychiatric Association, 2000

Brekke JS: An examination of the relationships among three outcome scales in schizophrenia. J Nerv Ment Dis 180:162–167, 1992

Coulehan J, Schulberg H, Block M, et al: Treating depressed primary care patients improves their physical, mental, and social functioning. Arch Intern Med 157:1113–1120, 1997

Dohrenwend BS, Dohrenwend BP, Link B, et al: Social functioning of psychiatric patients in contrast with community cases in the general population. Arch Gen Psychiatry 40:1174–1182, 1983

Dufton BD, Siddique CM: Measures in the day hospital. I. The Global Assessment of Functioning Scale. Int J Partial Hosp 8:41–49, 1992

Federal Register: Definition of Adults with a serious mental illness. Washington, DC, Office of the Federal Register, National Archives and Records Administration, 1993, vol 58, no 96, pp 29425

Fernando T, Mellsop G, Nelson K, et al: The reliability of Axis V of DSM-III. Am J Psychiatry 143:752–755, 1986

First MB, Spitzer RL, Gibbon M, et al: User's Guide for the Structured Clinical Interview for DSM-IV Axis I Disorders—Clinician Version (SCID-CV). Washington, DC, American Psychiatric Press, 1997

Goldman HH, Skodol AE, Lave TR: Revising Axis V for DSM-IV: a review of measures of social functioning. Am J Psychiatry 149:1148–1156, 1992

Government Performance Results Act of 1993, Pub. L. No. 103-62

Hall RCW: Global Assessment of Functioning: a modified scale. Psychosomatics 36:267–275, 1995

Howes JL, Haworth H, Reynolds P, et al: Outcome evaluation of a short-term mental health day treatment program. Can J Psychiatry 42:502–508, 1997

Johnston M, Pollard B: Consequences of disease: testing the WHO International Classification of Impairments, Disabilities, and Handicaps (ICIDH) model. Soc Sci Med 53:1261–1273, 2001

Loevdahl H, Friis S: Routine evaluation of mental health: reliable information or worthless "guesstimates"? Acta Psychiatr Scand 93:125–128, 1996

McLellan AT, Kushner H, Metzger D, et al: The fifth edition of the Addiction Severity Index. J Subst Abuse Treat 9:199–213, 1992

Moos R, McCoy L, Moos B: Global Assessment of Functioning (GAF) ratings: determinants and role as predictors of 1-year service use and treatment outcome. J Clin Psychol 56:449–461, 2000

Moos R, Nichol A, Moos B: Global Assessment of Functioning (GAF) ratings and the allocation and outcome of mental health care. Psychiatr Serv 53:730–737, 2002

Mueser KT, Becker DR, Torrey WC, et al: Work and nonvocational domains of functioning in persons with severe mental illness: a longitudinal analysis. J Nerv Ment Dis 185:419–426, 1997

National Advisory Mental Health Council (NAMHC): Health care reform for Americans with severe mental illness: report of the National Advisory Mental Health Council. Am J Psychiatry 150:1447–1465, 1993

Ouimette PC, Finney JW, Moos R: Twelve-step and cognitive-behavioral treatment for substance abuse: a comparison of treatment effectiveness. J Consult Clin Psychol 65:230–240, 1997

Patterson DA, Lee M: Field trial of the Global Assessment of Functioning scale–modified. Am J Psychiatry 152:1386–1388, 1995

Piersma HL, Boes JL: Agreement between patient self-report and clinician rating: concurrence between the BSI and the GAF among psychiatric inpatients. J Clin Psychol 51:153–157, 1995

Robert P, Aubin V, Dumarcet M, et al: Effect of symptoms on the assessment of social functioning: comparison between Axis V of DSM III-R and the Psychosocial Aptitude Rating Scale. Eur Psychiatry 6:67–71, 1991

Rosenheck R, DiLella D: Department of Veterans Affairs National Mental Health Program Performance Monitoring System: Fiscal Year 1998 Report. West Haven, CT, Northeast Program Evaluation Center (182), VA Connecticut Healthcare System, 1999

Roy-Byrne P, Dagadakis C, Unutzer J, et al: Evidence for limited validity of the revised Global Assessment of Functioning scale. Psychiatr Serv 47:864–866, 1996

Skodol AE, Link BG, Shrout PE, et al: Toward construct validity for DSM-III Axis V. Psychiatry Res 24:13–23, 1988

Stewart AL, Ware JE: Measuring Functioning and Well-Being: The Medical Outcomes Study Approach. Durham, NC, Duke University Press, 1992

Strauss JS, Carpenter WT: Prediction of outcome in schizophrenia. Arch Gen Psychiatry 34:159–163, 1977

Sullivan CW, Grubea JM: Who does well in a day treatment program? Following patients through 6 months of treatment. Int J Partial Hosp 7:101–110, 1991

Sullivan G, Dumenci L, Burnam A, et al: Validation of the Brief Instrumental Functioning Scale in a homeless population. Psychiatr Serv 52:1097–1099, 2001

U.S. Department of Veterans Affairs: Instituting Global Assessment of Functioning (GAF) scores in Axis V for mental health patients (VHA Directive 97-059). Washington, DC, U.S. Department of Veterans Affairs, 1997

Van Gastel A, Schotte C, Maes M: The prediction of suicidal intent in depressed patients. Acta Psychiatr Scand 96:254–259, 1997

Veterans Healthcare Eligibility Reform Act of 1996, Pub. L. No. 104-262, sec 1706(b)(1)

Index

*Pages numbers in **boldface type** refer to tables or figures.*

Anxiety *(continued)*
  comorbidity of, omission of, in
      diagnosis, frequency of, 8
  and depression, comorbidity of,
      60–61
Anxiety disorder(s)
  diagnosis of, using SCID,
      reliability of, 22
  epidemiology of, MIDAS
      findings on, 34
  not otherwise specified,
      prevalence of, **38**, 42
    with SCID *versus* clinical
        sample, **44**
  prevalence of, **38**
    with SCID *versus* clinical
        sample, 43, **44**
Asian Americans, psychiatric
    diagnoses for, accuracy of, 11
Attention-deficit/hyperactivity
    disorder, in children and
    adolescents
  diagnosis of
    using DISC, **82, 84, 86**
    using Voice DISC, **91**
  prevalence of, **41**
    with SCID *versus* clinical
        sample, **46**
Axis I psychopathology
  clinical epidemiology of,
      37–42
  as comorbid disorder, 37–42,
      38–41
    in body dysmorphic
        disorder, 36–37
    in borderline personality
        disorder, 49–51, **51**
    in depression, diagnosis of,
        study of, in MIDAS
        project, 48–49
  diagnosis of, MIDAS findings
      on, 42–43, **43**
  diagnostic criteria for,
      evaluation of, 54
  prevalence of, 37, **38–41**

  with SCID *versus* clinical
      sample, 43, **44–46**
  as principal diagnosis, 37–42,
      38–41
  screening for, 54. *See also*
      Psychiatric Diagnostic
      Screening Questionnaire
  self-report assessment for, 31

Beck's Lethality Rating Scale, xx,
    114
Behavior
  cultural context of, 9–10
  factors affecting, 9
  social context of, 9–10
  suicidal. *See* Suicidal behavior
Bias
  age-related, 12–13
  in diagnosis, xii, 10
Bipolar I disorder
  comorbidity of, in borderline
      personality disorder, 49
  prevalence of, **38**
    with SCID *versus* clinical
        sample, **44**
Bipolar II disorder
  comorbidity of, in borderline
      personality disorder, 49
  prevalence of, **38**
    with SCID *versus* clinical
        sample, **44**
Body dysmorphic disorder
  characteristics and correlates
      of, MIDAS findings on,
      36–37
  and depression, 37
  level of functioning in, 37
  prevalence of, **40**
    in outpatient psychiatric
        setting, 36
    with SCID *versus* clinical
        sample, **45**
  suicide risk in, 36–37
  treatment-seeking in, 52
  underdiagnosis of, 36–37

Composite International
Diagnostic Interview–
Primary Health Care Version,
diagnoses made using, and
primary care physicians'
diagnoses, comparison of, 5
Computer-assisted diagnostic
interview, 79–80. *See also*
Computerized Diagnostic
Interview Schedule for
Children
diagnoses made with
accuracy of, 4
and clinical diagnosis,
comparison of, 35
effect on clinical services,
92–95
socially sensitive material
reported on, 90–92
use of, 17–18
Computerized Diagnostic
Interview Schedule for
Children, xii, xix, 87–88
advantages of, 94–95
effect on clinical services,
94–95
Conduct disorder, diagnosis of
using DISC, **82, 84, 86**
using Voice DISC, **91,** 92
Cost-effectiveness, of
standardized assessment,
xii–xiii, xix, 19
Culture
effects on diagnostic accuracy,
xvi, 9–12
and psychiatric diagnostic
process, 13–14
Culture-bound disorders, 14
Cutoff scores, for diagnostic
instruments, 58–59

Deception, in psychiatric
diagnostic process, 13
Decision-making algorithms, for
psychiatric diagnosis, 18, 19

Delusion(s), presence/absence
of, assessment of, accuracy
of, 4
Delusional disorder, prevalence
of, **39**
with SCID *versus* clinical
sample, **45**
Depression
and anxiety, comorbidity of,
60–61
in children and adolescents,
diagnosis of
using DISC, **82, 84, 86**
using Voice DISC, **91,** 92
clinical epidemiology of, 37
comorbidity in, diagnosis of
breadth of assessment and,
49, **50**
study of, in MIDAS project,
48–49
comorbidity of
in body dysmorphic
disorder, 37
in borderline personality
disorder, 49
diagnosis of, 30
factors affecting, 14
by primary care physicians,
accuracy of, 4–5
using SCID, 60
diagnostic criteria for,
evaluation of, 54
epidemiology of, MIDAS
findings on, 34
prevalence of, **38**
with SCID *versus* clinical
sample, **44**
psychotic subtype of, and
PTSD, association of,
51–52
and suicide risk, 106,
107–108
treatment of, research on,
62–63, **64**
treatment-seeking in, 52

Family History Research
Diagnostic Criteria (FH-RDC),
in MIDAS project, 32
Fort Bragg Demonstration Project
on comorbidity of substance
abuse, 8

GAD. *See* Generalized anxiety
disorder
GAF scale. *See* Global Assessment
of Functioning scale
Gambling, pathological. *See*
Pathologic gambling
Generalized anxiety disorder
in children and adolescents,
diagnosis of
using DISC, **86**
using Voice DISC, **91,** 92
and mood disorders,
comorbidity of, 60–61
prevalence of, **38**
with SCID *versus* clinical
sample, **44**
treatment-seeking in, 52
Generic (Epidemiological)
DISC-IV, 84–87
reliability of, 85–87, **86**
Global Assessment of Functioning
scale, xiii
as outcome measure
preliminary analysis of,
141–146
systemwide implementation
of, xxi–xxii, 131–151
ratings on
in body dysmorphic
disorder, 37
compared with other
measures of functioning,
xxii, 146–148
as outcome predictor, xxii,
146, 149
relation to diagnosis and
symptom severity, xxii,
146–148

reliability of, xxii, 146–147, 149
and service utilization, xxii,
146, 148–149
as severity indicator, xxii, 131–151
systemwide implementation of,
xxi, 131–151
method for, 132–135, **134**
rationale for, 131–132
staff involvement in,
135–140
use of, training for, 135–137
national, by satellite
broadcast, 140–141
Gold standard diagnosis, in
Diagnostic Update Project, 6

5-HIAA. *See* 5-Hydroxyindoleacetic
acid
Hopelessness Scale, xx, 117–118
5-Hydroxyindoleacetic acid, CSF
levels of, and suicidal
behavior, 107–108
Hypochondriasis, prevalence of, **40**
with SCID *versus* clinical
sample, **45**

IDD. *See* Inventory to Diagnose
Depression
Impulse control disorder(s)
not otherwise specified,
prevalence of, **40**
with SCID *versus* clinical
sample, **46**
prevalence of, **40**
with SCID *versus* clinical
sample, 43, **46**
Impulsivity
CSF levels of 5-HIAA and, 108
and suicide risk, 106, 108
Intake evaluation, functions of, 68
Intermittent explosive disorder
prevalence of, **40**
with SCID *versus* clinical
sample, **46**
treatment-seeking in, 52

Interview(s). *See also* Computer-
assisted diagnostic interview
research diagnostic, 30, 54
semistructured, 78
advantages of, 80
for assessment of personality
disorders, 30
standardized, for research, 30
structured diagnostic, 78–80.
See also Diagnosis, using
structured assessment
advantages of, 80
cautions with, 22–23
for children, 75–96. *See also*
Diagnostic Interview
Schedule for Children
computerized, 79–80
in epidemiological studies,
33–42, 78
implementation of, xvi,
22–24, 79
traditional methods for
accuracy of diagnoses made
with, 4
problems with, 42, 76–77
unstructured
missed diagnoses with, 42
problems with, 76–77
Intoxication, acute, and suicide
risk, 106
Inventory to Diagnose
Depression, 54

Kleptomania, prevalence of, **40**
with SCID *versus* clinical
sample, **46**
K-SADS. *See* Schedule for
Affective Disorders and
Schizophrenia for School-
Aged Children

Labeling of patients, diagnoses
and, 2–3
Latinos, psychiatric diagnoses for,
accuracy of, 11

Lethality Scale, xx, 114
Longitudinal expert, all data
(LEAD) procedure, 18

Major depressive disorder. *See*
Depression
Marijuana abuse/dependence, in
children and adolescents,
diagnosis of, using Voice
DISC, **91**
MDD (major depressive disorder).
See Depression
MIDAS. *See* Rhode Island
Methods to Improve
Diagnostic Assessment and
Services
Miscommunication, in psychiatric
diagnostic process, 13
Mood disorders
comorbidity of, omission of,
in diagnosis, frequency
of, 8
diagnosis of, using SCID,
reliability of, 22
prevalence of, **38**
with SCID *versus* clinical
sample, 43, **44**
as principal diagnosis, 42

Negative predictive value, of
diagnostic instruments, 58
Nicotine dependence, in children
and adolescents, diagnosis
of, using Voice DISC,
91, 92
No-harm contract, and suicide
prevention, 109
Nosology, psychiatric
examination of, in MIDAS
project, 60–61
training of physicians in,
20–21
Nursing home population,
diagnostic assessment of,
accuracy of, 12–13

Psychiatric Diagnostic Screening
Questionnaire *(continued)*
diagnostic performance of, 57–60
initial development of, 54–57
revision of, 55–56
sensitivity of, 57–59
specificity of, 57–59
subscales of, 56–57
validation of, 55–57
Psychosocial crisis, and suicide
risk, 106
Psychotic disorder(s)
comorbidity of
in childhood trauma victims,
51
in PTSD, 51
diagnosis of
accuracy of, 10, 11
factors affecting, 14
structured methods for,
agreement among, 23
using SCID, reliability of, 22
not otherwise specified,
prevalence of, **39**
with SCID *versus* clinical
sample, **45**
prevalence of, **39**
with SCID *versus* clinical
sample, 43, **45**

Questionnaire(s). *See also*
Psychiatric Diagnostic
Screening Questionnaire; Self-
report assessment
and diagnostic interviews
comparison of, 79
level of agreement between, 53
in diagnostic screening, 53

Race, effects on diagnostic
accuracy, xvi, 9–13
Reasons for Living Inventory, xx,
118–119
Retirement status, and detection
of mental illness, 14

Rhode Island Methods to Improve
Diagnostic Assessment and
Services, xii, xvii–xviii, 29–68
components of, 31
epidemiologic findings in,
33–42
examination of nosologic issues
in, 60–61
methods of, 32–33
results from, 33–52
screening instrument
developed in, 52–60. *See
also* Psychiatric Diagnostic
Screening Questionnaire
treatment research in,
generalizability of, 62–63,
64
unanswered questions from,
63–68

Scale for Suicide Ideation, xx, 115
Schedule for Affective Disorders
and Schizophrenia for School-
Aged Children, 78, 80
Schizoaffective disorder,
prevalence of, **39**
with SCID *versus* clinical
sample, **45**
Schizophrenia
diagnosis of, accuracy of, 10, 11
patients with, communication
of diagnosis to, 15
prevalence of, **39**
with SCID *versus* clinical
sample, **45**
and suicide risk, 107
SCID. *See* Structured Clinical
Interview for DSM
Screening, psychiatric
diagnostic, instrument for. *See
also* Psychiatric Diagnostic
Screening Questionnaire
clinical need for, 52–60
in emergency room, 20–21
in primary care settings, 19–20

Self-report assessment. *See also*
Computerized Diagnostic
Interview Schedule for
Children; Psychiatric
Diagnostic Screening
Questionnaire
as adjunct to unstructured
interview, 67
for Axis I psychopathology, 31
in diagnostic screening, 53
Sensitivity, of diagnostic
instruments, 57–59
Separation anxiety, in children
and adolescents, diagnosis of
using DISC, **84, 86**
using Voice DISC, **91,** 92
Sex, of patient, and diagnostic
accuracy, 11
Sexual behavior, adolescent,
disclosure of, in computerized
self-assessment, 91
SIDP. *See* Structured Interview for
DSM-III Personality
Disorders
SIDP-IV. *See* Structured Interview
for DSM-IV Personality
Disorders
Social phobia
in children and adolescents,
diagnosis of
using DISC, **84, 86**
using Voice DISC, **91,** 92
clinical epidemiology of, 37–42
comorbidity of, in borderline
personality disorder, 49
diagnosis of, using SCID, 60
prevalence of, **38**
with SCID *versus* clinical
sample, **44**
treatment-seeking for, 52
Socioeconomic status, and
detection of mental illness, 14
Somatization
and detection of mental illness, 14
prevalence of, **40**

Somatoform disorder(s)
comorbidity of, in borderline
personality disorder, 49
not otherwise specified,
prevalence of, **40**
with SCID *versus* clinical
sample, **45**
prevalence of, **40**
with SCID *versus* clinical
sample, 43, **45**
Specificity, of diagnostic
instruments, 57–59
Specific phobia
in children and adolescents,
diagnosis of
using DISC, **86**
using Voice DISC, **91**
comorbidity of, in borderline
personality disorder, 49
prevalence of, **38,** 42
with SCID *versus* clinical
sample, **44**
treatment-seeking for, 52
Stereotyping, of people with
mental illness, 2–3
Structured Clinical Interview for
DSM
administration of, 22–23
training programs for, 23–24
in Diagnostic Update Project,
17–18
for DSM-III, accuracy of
diagnoses made with, 4
for DSM-IV, in MIDAS project, 31
for DSM-IV Axis I disorders
Clinician Version, 21
diagnoses using
and clinical diagnosis,
differences between,
xvi–xvii
follow-up interview after,
22
in MIDAS project, 32–33
nosologic issues raised by,
60–61

interrupted, definition of, 112–113

medical lethality of, assessment of, 117

precipitants of, 114

Suicide contagion, and suicide risk, 106

Suicide Intent Scale, xx, 116–117

Suicide-related behavior. *See* Suicidal behavior

Suicide risk
   assessment of, 106
      caveats for, 119
      clinical, 109–110
      components of, 119
      obstacles in, 109–110
      research, 110–119
      research *versus* clinical, 111–112
   in body dysmorphic disorder, 36–37
   detection of, xii–xiii, xix
   imminent, assessment of, 111
   lifetime, 111

Suicide scales, xx

Symptom(s)
   assessment of
      by emergency room physicians, accuracy of, 9
      by primary care physicians, accuracy of, 9
      presence/absence of, assessment of, accuracy of, 4
   severity of
      and detection of mental illness, 14
      relation to GAF ratings, xxii, 146–148

Texas Department of Mental Health and Mental Retardation, and university-based research program, linkage of, 6

Therapeutic alliance, development of, structured interviews and, 32–33

Tic disorder, in children and adolescents, diagnosis of, using Voice DISC, **91,** 92

Time allotment, for diagnostic evaluation, 53, 55, 63

Training
   in GAF scale use, 135–137
   national, by satellite broadcast, 140–141
   of physicians, in psychiatric nosology, 20–21
   in SCID use, 23–24

Treatment research, generalizability of, 62–63, **64**

Treatment-seeking
   factors affecting, 34
   reasons for, 52

Trichotillomania, prevalence of, **40**
   with SCID *versus* clinical sample, **46**

Undifferentiated somatoform disorder, prevalence of, **40**
   with SCID *versus* clinical sample, **45**

University of Texas Southwestern Medical Center at Dallas, research program of, community mental health program, linkage of, 6

Veterans Affairs, U.S. Department of, nationwide implementation of GAF scale use. *See* Global Assessment of Functioning scale

Violence, adolescent, disclosure of, in computerized self-assessment, 91

Voice DISC, xix, 88–89
   psychometric performance of, 89–90, **91**